Food Microbiology and Food Safety

Series Editor:
Michael P. Doyle

Food Microbiology and Food Safety Series

The Food Microbiology and Food Safety series is published in conjunction with the International Association for Food Protection, a non-profit association for food safety professionals. Dedicated to the life-long educational needs of its Members, IAFP provides an information network through its two scientific journals (Food Protection Trends and Journal of Food Protection), its educational Annual Meeting, international meetings and symposia, and interaction between food safety professionals.

Series Editor

Michael P. Doyle, *Regents Professor and Director of the Center for Food Safety, University of Georgia, Griffin, GA, USA*

Editorial Board

Francis F. Busta, *Director, National Center for Food Protection and Defense, University of Minnesota, Minneapolis, MN, USA*
Patricia Desmarchelier, *Food Safety Consultant, Brisbane, Australia*
Jeffrey Farber, *Bureau of Microbial Hazards, Ottawa, ON, Canada*
David Golden, *Professor of Microbiology, Department of Food Science and Technology, University of Tennessee, Knoxville, TN, USA*
Vijay Juneja, *Supervisory Lead Scientist, USDA-ARS, Philadelphia, PA, USA*

More information about this series at http://www.springer.com/series/7131

Frank Yiannas

Food Safety = Behavior

30 Proven Techniques to Enhance
Employee Compliance

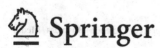
Springer

Frank Yiannas
Bentonville, AR, USA
www.foodsafetyculture.com

Food Microbiology and Food Safety
ISBN 978-1-4939-4395-1   ISBN 978-1-4939-2489-9   (eBook)
DOI 10.1007/978-1-4939-2489-9

Springer New York Heidelberg Dordrecht London
© Springer Science+Business Media New York 2015, Corrected at 2nd printing 2016
Softcover reprint of the hardcover 1st edition 2015

Printed on acid-free paper

Springer Science+Business Media LLC New York is part of Springer Science+Business Media (www.springer.com)

*This book is dedicated to my wife
and daughter, Diane Yiannas and Virginia
Yiannas Jones, for their love, support,
and kindness. They have been a blessing
to me and they have made me a better man.*

Contents

1 48 Million Versus One 1
Invoking Compassion to Give 1
What Does This Mean to Food Safety? 2

2 Getting Your Foot in the Door for Food Safety 5
Decreasing Restaurant Reservation Cancelations and No-Shows 6
Initial Safe Driver Commitment Influences Future Behavior 6
What Does This Mean for Food Safety? 7

3 Enclothed Food Safety? 9
What You Wear Influences What You Do 9
What Does This Mean to Food Safety? 10

4 Does What You See Influence What You Do? 13
Effect of Seeing Others Wear Personal Protective Equipment 13
What Does This Mean to Food Safety? 14

5 Priming the Pump for Enhanced Food Safety 15
Learning from Carwash Loyalty Cards 15
Reluctance to Waste or Perceived Progress? 16
What Does This Mean to Food Safety? 16

6 Influence Values to Change Attitudes 19
Affirmative Action Versus Equality 19
What Does This Mean to Food Safety? 20

7 Broken Windows and Food Safety 23
Broken Windows Theory 23
Car Vandalism and the Birth of the Theory 24
Graffiti's Influence on Other Behaviors 24
What Does This Mean to Food Safety? 24

8   **Learning from the Right Way or Wrong Way?**...................................   27
    Why Experience Matters...   27
    The Science of Training: What Really Works?.....................................   28
    What Training Firefighters Can Teach Us..   28
    What Does This Mean to Food Safety?...   29

9   **Make Food Safety the Social Norm**...   31
    Pointing and Gawking Experiment..   31
    Solomon Asche Experiment...   32
    Well Intentioned, Poorly Communicated...   32
    Making Hand Washing the Social Norm   33
    What Does This Mean to Food Safety?...   33

10 **Shining a Light on Food Safety**..   35
    The Difference Eight Light Bulbs Can Make   36
    What Does This Mean to Food Safety?...   36

11 **What Nouns, Verbs, & Voting Can Teach Us About Food Safety**.......   39
    Enhancing Voter Turnout   39
    What Does This Mean to Food Safety?...   40

12 **Birds of a Feather Might Influence Food Safety for Better**   41
    Homophily   41
    Principle of Likeness..   42
    Likeness and Adoption of Health-Related Behaviors............................   42
    What Does This Mean to Food Safety?...   43

13 **Keep Food Safety in Mind by Making It Rhyme**...............................   45
    Age-Old Tradition..   45
    Rhyming Helps Us Remember   45
    Poetic Effect on Believability   46
    What Does This Mean to Food Safety?...   47

14 **Making Scents of Food Safety**..   49
    Willingness to Help Others..   49
    Aromas and Safe Driving...   50
    What Does This Mean to Food Safety?...   50

15 **Font Style & Food Safety**   53
    Ease of Readability Matters...   54
    What Does This Mean to Food Safety?...   54

16 **Can SOPs Actually Hinder Food Safety?**   57
    If It's Hard to Read, It Must Be Hard to Do   58
    What Does This Mean to Food Safety?...   58

17 **Which One is Better, Written or Verbal?**..   59
    Method of Communication and Deception..   59
    E-Mail Versus Other Forms of Written Communication.........................   60
    What Does This Mean to Food Safety?...   61

18   Three Degrees of Food Safety 63
      People Do What Other People Do 63
      Three Degrees of Influence 64
      What Does this Mean to Food Safety? 64

19   Food Safety @ the Speed of Thought 67
      Thinking Fast & Risk Taking Behavior 67
      What Does this Mean to Food Safety? 68

20   Do Text Based Warning Labels Work? 71
      Changing Smoking Behaviors 71
      Graphic Cigarette Warning Labels 72
      What Does This Mean For Food Safety? 72

21   Enhancing Food Safety by Melody 75
      Music Affects Our Attitudes, Emotions, and Perceptions 75
      Background Music and Safe Driving Behaviors 76
      What Does This Mean to Food Safety? 77

22   Can the Words We Use Influence Risk Perception? 79
      Hard or Easy to Pronounce Fictitious Food Additives 79
      What Does This Mean to Food Safety? 80

23   Don't Be a Food Safety Bystander 81
      Willingness to Help in a Medical Emergency 81
      Where There Is Smoke, There Is Fire 82
      What Does This Mean to Food Safety? 82

24   To Checklist or Not to Checklist? 85
      Checklists Improve Healthcare Outcomes 85
      Lessons Learned from the Cockpit 86
      What Does This Mean to Food Safety? 87

25   The Most Powerful Word in Food Safety 89
      Moving to the Head of the Line 89
      What Does This Mean to Food Safety? 90

26   Food Safety in Mind through Building Design 93
      Influencing Behavior by Design 93
      Collective Effects of Building Intent 93
      What Does This Mean to Food Safety? 94

27   Does How You Make a Food Safety Request Matter? 97
      What Does This Mean to Food Safety? 98

28   Is the Sum of Food Safety Efforts Greater Than In Parts? 99
      What Does This Mean to Food Safety? 100

29   Making Food Safety Fun 101
      The Fun Theory 101
      The World's Deepest Garbage Bin 101

Positive Consequences Eat Negative Ones for Lunch 102
What Does This Mean to Food Safety? 103

30 Role Modeling Food Safety 105
Influencing Others to Wash Their Hands 105
More Hand Wash Sinks or More Role Models 106
The Findings 106
What Does This Mean to Food Safety? 107

Conclusion 109

Acknowledgment 111

References 113

Introduction

As a food safety professional, getting others to comply with what you are asking them to do is critical, but it is not easy. In fact, it can be very hard to change other's behaviors. And if you are like most food safety professionals, you have probably received little or no formal training on how to influence or change people's behaviors.

But what if I told you that simple and proven behavioral science techniques exist, and, if applied strategically, can significantly enhance your ability to influence others and improve food safety. Would you be interested?

The need to better integrate the important relationship between behavioral science and food safety is what motivated me to write this book, *Food Safety = Behavior, 30 Proven Techniques to Enhance Employee Compliance*.

When it comes to food safety, people's attitudes, choices, and behaviors are some of the most important factors that influence the overall safety of our food supply. Real-world examples of how these human factors influence the safety of our food range from whether or not a food worker will decide to wash his or her hands before working with food to the methods a health department utilizes while attempting to improve food safety compliance within a community to the decisions a food manufacturer's management team will make on how to control a food safety hazard. They all involve human elements.

If concepts related to human and social behavior are so important to advancing food safety, why are they noticeably absent or lacking in the food safety profession today? Although there are probably several good reasons, I believe it is largely due to the fact that, historically, food safety professionals have not received adequate training or education in the behavioral sciences. Therefore, there are numerous food safety professionals who approach their jobs with an over-reliance on the food sciences alone. They rely too heavily, in my opinion, on traditional food safety approaches based on training, inspections, and testing.

Despite the fact that thousands of employees have been trained in food safety around the world, millions of dollars have been spent globally on food safety research, and countless inspections and tests have been performed at home and abroad, food safety remains a significant public health challenge. Why is that? The answer to this question reminds me of a quote by the late psychologist Abraham Maslow, who said, *"If the only tool you have is a hammer, you tend to see every problem as a nail."* To improve food safety, we have to realize that it's more than just food science; it's the behavioral sciences too.

Think about it. If you are trying to improve the food safety performance of an organization, industry, or region of the world, what you are really trying to do is change peoples' behaviors. *Simply put, food safety equals behavior.* This truth is the fundamental premise upon which this entire book is based.

How does one effectively influence the behaviors of a worker, a social group, a community, or an organization?

While it is not easy, fortunately, there is good news for today's more progressive, behavior-based food safety professional. Over the past 50 years, an incredible amount of research has been done in the behavioral and social sciences that have provided valuable insights into the thoughts, attitudes, and behaviors of humans. Applying these studies' conclusions to our field has the potential to dramatically change our preventative food safety approaches, enhance employee compliance, and, most importantly, save lives.

One of the most exciting aspects of behavioral science research is that its results are often of simple and practical use to numerous professions, including ours – food safety. Generally, the principles learned through behavioral science research require little technical or scientific equipment to implement. They usually do not require large expenses. What is required, however, is an understanding of the research data and the ability to infer how the research might be used to solve a problem in your area of concern.

In this book, *Food Safety = Behavior*, I've decided to collect some of the most interesting behavioral science studies I've reviewed over the past few years, which I believe might have relevance to food safety. I've assembled them into one easy-to-use book with suggested applications in how they might be used to advance food safety.

To get the most out of this book, at the end of each chapter, I strongly encourage you to spend a few minutes thinking about the behavioral science principle you have just read, what it means to food safety, and how you might apply that principle in your own organization (or in your role) to improve food safety. For those in academic settings, you might also want to make a list of potential questions for further research.

In summary, this book is devoted to introducing you to new ideas and concepts that have not been thoroughly reviewed, researched, and, more importantly, applied in the field of food safety. It is my attempt to arm you with new behavioral science tools to further reduce food safety risks in certain parts of the food system and world. I am convinced that we need to adopt new, out-of-the-box thinking that is more heavily focused on influencing and changing human behavior in order to accomplish this goal.

It is my hope that by simply reading this book, you pick up a few good ideas, tips, or approaches that can help you improve the food safety performance of your organization or area of responsibility. If you do, I will consider this book a success.

In closing, thanks for taking the time to read *Food Safety = Behavior* and, more importantly, for all that you are doing to advance food safety, so that people worldwide can live better.

Frank

If you have any questions, comments, or suggestions, I would love to hear from you. You can e-mail me at foodsafetyculture@msn.com or follow me on twitter @frankyiannas.

Chapter 1
48 Million Versus One

As a food safety professional, I'm sure you have a good grasp on the latest food-borne disease statistics published by the Centers for Disease Control and Prevention (CDC). According to the CDC, approximately 48 million Americans experience a foodborne illness annually. Of these, 138,000 require hospitalization and, tragically, around 3,000 die.

While, to me, these statistics are alarming, what do you think they mean to the average person or employee? When they are presented, as is often the case in food safety training classes, do you think it fills others with compassion and motivates them to work in a safer manner to reduce the chances of another outbreak and prevent more foodborne victims? You might find the answer to this question to be counter-intuitive.

If I told you that trying to persuade others on the importance of food safety by talking about the 48 million cases of foodborne illness annually may be less effective than talking about just one, would you believe me?

Invoking Compassion to Give

Previous research by Small and Loewenstein (2003) investigated whether a person's motivation or compassion to give would change if they were told the personal details of just one victim, perhaps a child, as compared to a larger group of unidentified victims. Their research demonstrated that people tend to give more money to causes with identifiable victims, such as "Baby Jessica" who fell down a well in 1987, rather than to causes with unknown victims, such as the thousands of starving children in an under-developed country.

In an advancement of this initial study, Small et al. (2007) wanted to know whether educating people about this "discrepancy principle" (the increased likelihood to give to an identified person vs. a larger group), would increase giving to statistical

© Springer Science+Business Media New York 2015

F. Yiannas, *Food Safety = Behavior*, Food Microbiology and Food Safety,
DOI 10.1007/978-1-4939-2489-9_1

groups of unidentified people or decrease giving to a single identified victim. In short, they wondered if people could be taught to "value life consistently."

In a series of experiments, they approached students in a student union and asked them to participate in a survey in exchange for $5.00. At the end of the survey, each participant was given the opportunity to donate any portion of their $5.00 to *Save the Children*, an organization that helps with severe starvation in Africa.

In experiment number one, students received statistical information about *Save the Children* and then were asked to donate. Half of them were given a brief description of the discrepancy principle before being asked to give and the other half were not. For this group, giving was about the same with and without the discrepancy information: ($1.26 vs. $1.17).

In experiment number two, students were asked to give to *Save the Children* following a presentation containing information about a starving little girl and her picture (rather than statistical information). Again, half of the people in this group were told about the discrepancy principle and the other half were not. Amazingly, when asked to give by simply presenting the story of one little girl, without knowledge of the discrepancy principle, the students' average giving jumped to $2.81! However, when presented with information of the discrepancy principle, student giving dropped to $1.36, in line with the amount given when presented with statistical information about the larger group.

For experiment number three, Small, Loewenstein, and Slovic wondered what would happen to students' willingness to give if they were presented with both statistical information and an identifiable victim, while being unaware of the discrepancy principle. In this experiment, they found that students were willing to give $2.38 when presented with the little girl's picture. However, when presented with both statistical information and the personal testimonial, students on average gave only $1.43, significantly less. In other words, even when an effective personal story of an identified individual was used, if students knew the statistics, they were not willing to give as much. In fact, on average, people gave $0.85 less!

What Does This Mean to Food Safety?

This research suggests that a common practice used by food safety professionals and trainers might be wrong or ineffective. When trying to persuade others to take food safety seriously, do not use statistics (i.e. 48 million cases of foodborne disease annually). Instead, put a face on food safety and tell a story using a real-world example of a victim of foodborne disease. Research suggests that under this method, people are much more likely to be moved with compassion and act.

Moreover, even when attempting to influence others by telling the story of an individual who suffered the tragic consequences of a severe case of foodborne disease, it appears that you should not mention the statistical information about the millions of other cases of foodborne disease annually. It could do more harm than good.

What does this research not tell us? It does not address whether we should have a "poster child" victim for every type of foodborne illness or a single victim in general. We also do not know whether we should present new victims of the same illness over time, or whether we should emphasize one victim's story for years.

Think about these research findings and how it might be applied to food safety. While I am sure you can think of many creative ways in how you might use this research, let me illustrate a few ideas to consider.

- Do a thorough review of all of your organization's food safety training and education modules. How many times do you use statistics in them to make your point versus a powerful testimonial? The results of this exercise might surprise you. In many organizations, I have found that this principle's use is completely missing in well intended food safety training and educational approaches.
- When training employees about the importance of food allergies, instead of teaching the class about the number of Americans with food allergies, tell one of the many documented stories, in detail, of a child that tragically died due to unknowingly consuming an undeclared allergen present in food, because of an error in practice that resulted in cross-contact.

In closing, think about the findings of this research, its implications, and how you might apply it to your daily work. Remember, people are much more likely to be moved by a personal testimonial, not a statistic.

Chapter 2
Getting Your Foot in the Door for Food Safety

If I told you that there was a simple behavioral science technique that, if applied strategically, could significantly enhance your ability to influence others to comply with your requests, would you be interested?

Whether it's trying to influence key leaders in the organization to be more supportive of food safety or getting front-line employees to comply with certain requests, such as washing their hands or taking food temperatures – *food safety equals behavior*. As I have stated before, if you think you are going to achieve behavior change by solely focusing on conducting audits and training, I can guarantee you, you will not succeed. Remember, human behavior is more complex than this. You will need more than audits, training, and a reliance on the food sciences to be successful.

According to best-selling author and psychologist Dr. Robert Cialdini (1993), people want to behave in a way that is consistent with their values, beliefs, and/or commitments. In other words, once a person has made a choice or taken a position on a matter, they will want to behave in a manner that's consistent with that commitment. And if a person has stated their beliefs publically, or if they have made a verbal (or better yet a written) commitment to an idea or goal, their behaviors are much more likely to be consistent with their stated beliefs or commitments.

What causes this behavior? According to behavioral scientists, in general, people do not want to be known as liars or wishy-washy. Instead, they prefer to be known as consistent, trustworthy, and true to themselves. Inconsistency is a socially undesirable trait.

Let me provide a couple of studies that illustrate just how powerful this principle can be in influencing others' behavior.

© Springer Science+Business Media New York 2015
F. Yiannas, *Food Safety = Behavior*, Food Microbiology and Food Safety,
DOI 10.1007/978-1-4939-2489-9_2

Decreasing Restaurant Reservation Cancelations and No-Shows

A Chicago restaurant owner was having trouble with "no shows." People would make dinner reservations, but fail to appear for dinner. Additionally, they would not call to cancel their reservations. At this restaurant, it was common for the host or hostess to take the reservation by phone and then say, "*please call if you change your plans.*" For months, the no-show rate at this restaurant was approximately 30 %.

As part of a behavioral science study, researchers thought that if they were able to get callers to make a commitment, the "no-show" rate might drop. Accordingly, they conducted a study, whereby, they instructed the receptionists to stop saying, "*Please call us if you change your plans,*" and start saying, "*Will you please call us if you change your plans?*" Furthermore, the receptionist was instructed to intentionally pause and wait for the caller to respond. Simply put, the receptionist was asked to make two small changes that required little to no effort and certainly no new costs. First, they modified what they said to callers by adding two small words to the beginning of the script – *will you*. Second, instead of ending the script with a period, they ended with a question mark, which made callers make a commitment – either yes or no.

What do you think happened by simply adding two words to the script and ending with a question mark? Amazingly, by making these simple and almost effortless changes, the no-show rate at this restaurant dropped a whopping 20 % points from 30 % to 10 %.

As yet another powerful example of how people, in general, desire to be consistent with previous commitments they have made, let me share a study that illustrates what behavioral scientists call the "foot-in-the-door technique" to getting others to say yes to subsequent requests.

Initial Safe Driver Commitment Influences Future Behavior

Freedman and Fraser (1966) wanted to test their assumption that once people committed to a smaller request, they are much more likely to comply with a larger, related request. To do so, they conducted a series of creative experiments involving people who lived in an affluent neighborhood in California. Residents in the neighborhood were randomly divided into two groups.

In Group 1, an enterprising research student posing as a volunteer worker went door-to-door in the neighborhood asking the residents a preposterous question. They asked the homeowners if they would be willing to install a public-service billboard on their front lawn. To get an idea of the sign's design, they would show the homeowners a photo of a house that was largely blocked by a poorly lettered sign that read, DRIVE CAREFULLY. As you can imagine, the vast majority of home owners (83 %) refused to participate.

For Group 2, a research student posing as a volunteer worker once again went door-to-door asking homeowners to participate in a public-service promotion. However, this time, they asked homeowners a much simpler request. They asked if they would be willing to put up a small "3×3" sticker that read "*Be a safe driver*" in one of their front windows. Based on this much smaller request, most did. Three weeks later, the researchers sent back another student to these same homes with a different request. This time they asked homeowners if they would be willing to place a large public service billboard on their lawns. To give an idea of just how the sign would look, the student once again showed a photograph depicting an attractive house that was almost completely obscured from view by the large sign reading DRIVE CAREFULLY.

You might think that a majority, as in group 1, would not want such an eye-sore on their lawn. However, an astonishing 76 % of those who had put up the sticker agreed to have the huge sign placed on their lawns! In other words, compliance with this request jumped from 17 % in group 1 to a whopping 76 % in group 2.

Freedman and Fraser hypothesized that based on the principle of consistency, putting up the initial sticker (a foot-in-the-door) appears to have implanted the idea among homeowners to think of themselves as people who were active campaigners for public good and now – to be consistent – they eagerly complied to preserve that self image.

What Does This Mean for Food Safety?

The implications from this study are clear and amazing. By understanding and utilizing the principles of consistency and commitment, food safety professionals might be able to provoke a stronger response in those they are trying to influence and, ultimately, get them to comply more frequently with desired behaviors or bigger requests.

How might a food safety professional use this principle to enhance food safety? While I am sure you can think of many ways you might put this principle into practice, here is one good example.

In general, when front-line employees are trained in food safety, they are asked to sign a roster to prove that they have attended the training or click a completion button on a computer based learning (CBL) module. Why do compliance professionals do this? Usually, it's to ensure there is a record that can be used as proof that the organization has met its regulatory requirement that all of its food handlers are trained. However, by knowing about the principle of consistency, how might food safety professionals approach this differently? What if employees were asked at the end of such training to make a written (or electronic) *commitment* stating that they would adhere to the principles they learned in the training, do you think the class would be more effective at influencing their future behaviors? I do. And the research by Freedman and Fraser suggests it would too.

Remember, most people want to live up to their commitments, especially if it's in writing. By asking employees to commit to practicing the food safety tips they have learned, rather than just signing that they have completed the course, we are much more likely to pressure them to be consistent with the food safety principles they have just learned.

In closing, think about the principles of consistency and commitment and how they might be used to improve food safety. And remember, by getting your foot-in-the-door for food safety with a small initial request, you might just be opening up the door to influence desired food safety behaviors in a much greater way.

Chapter 3
Enclothed Food Safety?

Although I've always realized the importance of first impressions through the clothing a person wears, I've always thought the phrase – "dress for success" – was kind of shallow. But what if I told you that the way a person dresses might be more important than simply influencing the way others perceive them? It could also influence their behaviors. Would you believe me?

What You Wear Influences What You Do

Adam and Galinsky (2012), two behavioral science researchers, wanted to know the impact clothing had on behavior. They coined the phrase '*enclothed cognition*' to express their hypothesis that people's actions are affected by both "the symbolic meaning of the clothes" and whether they "actually wear them."

To test their hypothesis, they conducted a series of experiments.

In the first experiment, they brought undergraduate college students into a lab for a cognitive task. One group of students was asked to wear a lab coat during the task and the other group was not. The error rate of those who wore the lab coats was almost 50 % less than those that did not wear the lab coats. Put another way, those wearing street clothes had almost twice as many errors as those who wore a lab coat.

In order to determine whether their results were due to the mere thought of the lab coat or to the actual wearing of the coat, they designed a second experiment. This time, they divided the students into three groups:

1. Those that wore a lab coat, which was described as a "doctor's" coat
2. Those that wore the same lab coat, but this time it was described as an "artistic painter's" coat, and
3. Those that only saw a doctor's coat

Keep in mind that these coats were exactly the same, just described differently.

© Springer Science+Business Media New York 2015

F. Yiannas, *Food Safety = Behavior*, Food Microbiology and Food Safety,

DOI 10.1007/978-1-4939-2489-9_3

Amazingly, only those who actually wore the "doctor's coat" performed better. In other words, simply seeing the doctor's coat didn't affect performance any more than by wearing the artist's coat. They confirmed their findings by demonstrating that even subjects who identified with a doctor's coat by writing an essay about it did not perform as well as those that actually wore the coat.

Of importance, the researchers established that wearing the lab coat was associated with attentiveness, carefulness, responsibility, and a scientific focus. Thus, it was the actual wearing of the coat and the knowledge of its associations that caused the behavior change. They suggest that this research has broader implications. For example, how do other types of outfits such as a judge's robe, a firefighter's uniform, or a finely tailored business suit influence behavior? What attitudes and behaviors are associated with these uniforms? In addition, might this effect wear off over time or would it maintain its impact?

What Does This Mean to Food Safety?

The implications of this research are quite thought-provoking. While food safety professionals have always cared about the clothing worn by food employees, it has always been to prevent contamination of food, equipment, and utensils – not to influence behavior. However, this research suggests that the uniforms an employee wears might actually influence their attentiveness, carefulness, and responsibility when preparing food.

If you are like me, you were probably fascinated by the results of this study. And while you have probably seen "enclothed cognition" in action in other professions or areas of society, you may have never taken the time to reflect on its influence on human behavior. Think about airline pilots, military officers, and boy or girl scouts to name just a few. Do you think their behaviors change or are influenced by the clothes they wear? Of course they are.

Based on the results of this research, how do you think this principle might be used to further strengthen food safety? Here are a few things to consider.

- Are we putting enough thought into the dress code required of employees, and do we consider what it might mean to food safety, beyond simple cleanliness?
- Could compliance with desired food safety behaviors be improved by implying expected behaviors with particular articles of clothing? For example, can we create a "be food safe" apron or vest (similar in idea to the symbolic vests worn by school cross-guards), which implies that once you put on this garment there are expected behaviors a person must follow?
- Often times, there is an implied hierarchy by the clothing or uniforms required in different positions (management, hourly, etc.). Could there also be implied behaviors that vary depending on the position and clothing required of them?

- The researchers used a new, clean lab coat. Would the results have been different if it were a wrinkled, dirty, or stained lab coat?
- Lastly, if we have a laid back, wear whatever-you-want dress code, does this result in a lack of compliance with desired food safety behaviors?

Think about these findings and questions. We often expend great efforts to reduce error rates by just a few percentage points. However, in the Adam and Galinsky study, errors rates were reduced 50 % by simply changing the clothes people wore.

We often hear the phrase, "food safety: it's in your hands." But can it also be that food safety improves by the clothes we wear?

Chapter 4
Does What You See Influence What You Do?

Do the behaviors of others influence your behavior? Be honest. If you are like most people, you want to think that you are fairly independent: other's actions do not necessarily influence your own actions. However, if you pause to think about yourself, visual observations of others are important. If they were not important, companies would not spend millions of dollars annually on commercials depicting people like you using their products. As another example, examine the most recent high school dress fad. You have heard about it. Students see their favorite celebrity wearing something, imitate them in their own dress, and thus create the next fashion fad.

Effect of Seeing Others Wear Personal Protective Equipment

How about in the workplace? Are you influenced by what other workers do? Olson and others (2009) wanted to know just that. They evaluated how the varying percentages of personal protection equipment (PPE) used in a training video impacted the use of PPE by new employees who had seen the video. In other words, they wanted to know if varying the percentage compliance of PPE worn in a training video would influence actual PPE used by employees in a linear fashion. This idea is generally known as positive social modeling (rather than negative social modeling which would show what *not* to do). Of particular interest, this experiment did not involve interactions between people at all; it relied solely on visual observations via video.

For the study, the researchers recruited people to participate in a 'baggage screening experiment' in which they would use a computer to look for knives in baggage going through an x-ray scanner. Prior to running the program (or conducting the baggage screening), each participant was shown a training video of how to perform the task. In the video, three female workers were shown at computer terminals receiving instructions about the task. Beside each computer was a pair of yellow

© Springer Science+Business Media New York 2015
F. Yiannas, *Food Safety = Behavior*, Food Microbiology and Food Safety,
DOI 10.1007/978-1-4939-2489-9_4

earmuffs. The experimental conditions were manipulated by having one, two, or all three of the video trainees put on and wear the ear muffs while doing the task in the video. No mention of the earmuffs or safety equipment was made during the video, nor was there instruction given to the study participants concerning the ear muffs.

The room created for the study participants was set up much like it was in the training video, with a pair of earmuffs lying next to the computer. Additionally, there was a 70 decibel level of white noise playing in the background during the task. After watching the respective training video, each person worked on the bagged screening task for 40 min. Every 10 min, researchers observed whether the ear muffs were being worn by the study participants.

As the number of workers in the video using PPE increased from 0 of 3, to 1 of 3, to 2 of 3, to 3 of 3, the percentages of study participants which used PPE at least once during the 40 min task were 25 %, 19 %, 38 %, and 69 %.

Directionally, as the number of workers observed in the training video using PPE increased, the number of study participants who wore PPE also increased. The researchers speculate about the reason why PPE use was actually less for participants who observed 1 of 3 trainees wear PPE (19 %) versus those that observed none of the 3 trainees wear PPE (25 %). They suggest that seeing only 1 of 3 trainees use PPE may have resulted in negative reinforcement, i.e. participants observed that most of the trainees weren't wearing PPE and this led to reduced use. However, as observed PPE use increased, use among participants increased proportionally.

What Does This Mean to Food Safety?

The inferences from this study are clear and significant. Simply demonstrating the correct or desired behavior in training can influence behavior in the workplace. In addition, if compliance is proportional to the observed frequency of the desired behavior, then it is crucial to have as much of the desired behavior as possible modeled correctly for new employees. In other words, it is important to show the desired behavior as the social norm.

Of particular interest, the researchers did not mention the PPE in any way in either the research study or video. The effect on the participants was achieved simply by showing its use in an auxiliary fashion.

In closing, think about the application of this research and how it might apply to food safety training programs. We use a lot of training videos and video clips in the industry. Many of these videos often have a single individual demonstrating a desired behavior or task. Since this effect is based on the percentage of compliance by employees in the video, maybe we should consider reworking training materials to include more than one person demonstrating the desired behavior or task, and ensure all employees in the video performing the task correctly, using the proper gloves, etc. In other words, simply showing the desired behavior once as an instructional aide may not be enough. Instead, if your desire is not only to demonstrate skill but also to motivate the desired behavior, you have to show that the behavior is the social norm, followed by all employees.

Chapter 5
Priming the Pump for Enhanced Food Safety

What if I told you that I believe some food safety failures occur because organizations fail to even get started on making the changes they need to make in order to enhance food safety? They fail to overcome inertia to enact organizational change.

However, there's a behavioral principle that you can use, in some instances, to overcome this problem. In fact, coffee shop employees use this principle all the time. Before opening, they put a couple of dollars or a handful of change in a tip jar and place it in front of their register. This 'primes the pump' so to speak. Thus, as their first customers buy coffee, they are more inclined to leave a tip since someone else has already done so. In economics, the phrase "priming the pump" is used to describe pumping money into an economy in hopes of stimulating economic activity.

Learning from Carwash Loyalty Cards

Nunes and Drèze (2006) conducted an experiment to determine if this idea also works on consumers. In their first experiment, they handed out 300 loyalty cards at a carwash. Half of the cards they gave away required eight carwashes to earn a free car wash. The other half, called the "endowed" group, required ten carwashes to earn a free car wash, but two of the boxes were already stamped (i.e., they primed the pump). In other words, both groups of people had to purchase eight carwashes to receive a free car wash.

Despite both groups having the exact same requirement, what do you think actually happened? Interestingly, 34% of those who received the endowed cards purchased eight additional carwashes and redeemed them for a free car wash versus only 19% of those who began with a blank card. In both groups, the time period between carwashes decreased as they earned more stamps. However, those with the endowed cards purchased their first carwash 2.5 days sooner than those who began with a blank card. In summary, the researchers concluded that priming the pump for carwash users increased both the rate and speed of redemption (completion).

© Springer Science+Business Media New York 2015
F. Yiannas, *Food Safety = Behavior*, Food Microbiology and Food Safety,
DOI 10.1007/978-1-4939-2489-9_5

Reluctance to Waste or Perceived Progress?

In experiment two, the researchers wanted to determine why this effect exists. They believed that the phenomena was due either to a reluctance to waste the accumulation or to the perception of progress toward completion of the program. To figure this out, they set up a mock frequent buyer program for a campus restaurant. They manipulated both the percent of the endowment (either 2 of 12 or 5 of 15 complete) and the actual dollar value of the endowment.

They found that no significant difference existed between the values of the endowed amounts. This means that people were not more inclined toward the program because of how much money was endowed at the onset. This discovery also indicates that a reluctance to waste money was not the motivating factor.

However, those who were endowed with 5 out of 15 had a significantly higher evaluation of the program than those who were endowed with 2 out of 12, even though both groups would have to make the same number of purchases in the program. Thus, the researchers suggested that the motivating factor was the student's perceived progress toward completion of the program.

What Does This Mean to Food Safety?

The results of this research are clear. Starting a person with some progress towards the completion of a program increases their likelihood of completing the program while decreasing the amount of time it takes to do so.

What are the food safety implications of these findings? While I am sure you can think of a variety of ways in which you might apply it, let me give you a couple of examples worth considering.

- First, I think this principle could have a positive effect on the outcome of health inspections of food establishments. For example, if an establishment requires inspection four times a year, what if you began by automatically awarding one inspection out of five with an A? In this way, every establishment begins with an A toward its goal, while in actuality it leaves the number of required inspections they need to pass unchanged. Would establishments be more likely to strive to pass the four remaining inspections with acceptable grades? The results from these studies conducted by Nunes and Drèze suggest that they would.
- Second, consider the way certification bodies or standard owners score food safety audits. What if every organization that met a certain set of criteria knew that they automatically started with a portion of the overall potential points in their score. Even if the overall scoring scheme was manipulated so that the establishment still had to demonstrate the same level of conformance as before, the establishment would feel well on its way to passing the audit, and may work harder to ensure that it met the other requirements needed to pass the audit.

Think about other possibilities in which this principle might be used to enhance food safety. Could certifications, training programs, out-of-compliance rates, and incentive programs all benefit from this effect?

In closing, think, think, and think about potential applications. Remember, food safety equals behavior, and it is impossible to strengthen employee compliance with desired behaviors without change.

Chapter 6
Influence Values to Change Attitudes

Have you ever tried to change someone's attitude? If you have, you know it can be pretty tough. In fact, public health and food safety professionals try to change peoples' attitudes all the time in hopes of getting them to adopt safer behaviors or adhere to company policies and practices. Why? Because they know that a person's attitude on an issue can influence their behavior related to that topic. However, a growing body of research suggests that trying to directly influence a person's attitude can backfire, causing him or her to only strengthen their resolve in their current way of thinking.

Affirmative Action Versus Equality

Three behavioral scientists, Blankenship et al. (2012), wanted to investigate whether a better way exists to change a person's attitude without directly attacking their attitude on a topic. In other words, they wondered whether influencing or relating to a person's value system might in turn change their attitude towards a policy.

In this study, the researchers chose to evaluate whether changes in a person's opinion about the value of equality could in turn influence their attitude about the policy of affirmative action. In the experiment, 82 study participants (students at a mid-western college) were split into two groups. Researchers told one group that they would read an editorial piece about affirmative action (a policy) while the other group was told that they would read an editorial piece about equality (a value). However, the text given to both groups to read was identical. Before and after the reading, the groups were asked to rate their opinions toward affirmative action through a series of questions rated on a scale of 1–9 (1 = harmful; 9 = beneficial). The average score on affirmative action before the readings was the same for both groups.

© Springer Science+Business Media New York 2015   19
F. Yiannas, *Food Safety = Behavior*, Food Microbiology and Food Safety,
DOI 10.1007/978-1-4939-2489-9_6

As hypothesized by the researchers, participants that read the editorial piece they thought was on affirmative action did not change their attitudes much towards the policy. The group's average score on their attitude towards affirmative action changed by less than one point after reading the editorial piece (post-reading change=0.7). However, the participants that read the editorial piece they thought was on the value of equality had a significantly changed opinion towards affirmative action after reading the article (post-reading change=1.8). Remember, both groups read the same exact article!

The researchers concluded that attitudes towards affirmative action changed more when the information was presented as a message related to the *value* of equality as opposed to the exact same message being presented as a *policy* on affirmative action.

What Does This Mean to Food Safety?

The implications of this research are clear. If you are attempting to change the attitudes of front-line employees towards food safety by telling them that it is a company policy or a requirement by law to behave in a certain way, you may not be very persuasive. However, linking food safety requests to related-values or personal beliefs might be much more effective at causing a genuine change in an employee's attitude towards a topic.

It is important to note that additional studies on this subject have shown that there must be a link between the desired attitude and the value one is focused on influencing. Trying to influence a value that has no connection to an attitude does not produce a change.

As you think about how you might use this principle to enhance food safety, consider the following:

- What are the values that form the basis for how your company makes decisions? Are any of the organization's values related or linked to food safety in any way?
- If so, how can you clearly make the link between food safety and the company's value to strengthen attitudes among employees at all levels about the importance of food safety?
- For example, if a company states that one of their values is "respect" for their customers, one could say that "*it is because we respect our customers that we care about their safety.*" Making sure that employees know that food safety requests are related to the value of respect could strengthen their compliance with desired food safety behaviors and tasks.
- As yet another example, instead of trying to persuade restaurant owners to comply with the food code because it's the law, would health inspectors have more success by linking food safety to a related societal value and talking about food code compliance in that manner?

- Lastly, learn from other areas of life and other disciplines. For example, think about the many initiatives companies have today regarding environmental stewardship and sustainability. Many of these initiatives are not being driven in order to comply with environmental law. Instead, these companies are responding to the new societal norm (shared value) that is emerging in certain parts of the world with the realization that we must do more to take care of the environment.

In summary, remember that employees are not generally moved towards complying with food safety because it is the company's policy or the law. Link food safety to an underlying or related value and they will be much more likely to comply.

Chapter 7
Broken Windows and Food Safety

If I were to ask you what broken windows, the ex-mayor of New York City (Rudy Giuliani), and graffiti can teach us about food safety and sanitation, what would your answer be?

I suspect many would consider 9/11 and the great crisis management skills shown by the mayor and his New York City emergency management team. Although this is a good answer, it is not the one I am looking for. The answer to my question is quite different. It is about a behavioral science principle that I believe has direct relevance to food safety.

Broken Windows Theory

In 1982, social scientists James Wilson and George Kelling proposed what is now called the Broken Windows theory. This theory suggested that even small signs of disorder—such as a single broken window in a housing project or a storefront that goes unfixed—could encourage more widespread negative behavior in other areas, because of the social norms that its presence communicates. In the 1990s, New York city Mayor Rudy Giuliani, his police chief, and other city officials subscribed to this theory and started focusing their attention on combating small but powerful signs of disorder such as litter and petty crime. Accordingly, they began removing graffiti, sweeping streets, and enacting a "zero tolerance" policy for other destructive behavior that occurred in the city. It is believed that this zero-tolerance policy decreased acts of vandalism against city buildings, and brought about one of the greatest turnarounds in the city's history. As someone who traveled to New York during the 1980s and 1990s (and being born in Manhattan), I can remember the dramatic turnaround. It was incredible.

© Springer Science+Business Media New York 2015
F. Yiannas, *Food Safety = Behavior*, Food Microbiology and Food Safety,
DOI 10.1007/978-1-4939-2489-9_7

Car Vandalism and the Birth of the Theory

The broken window theory is reported to have been originally based on the work by Philip Zimbardo, a Stanford psychologist, but has been proven many times over in a variety of experiments. In Zimbardo's social psychological experiment, he arranged to have an automobile without license plates parked with its hood up on a street in the Bronx and a comparable automobile on a street in Palo Alto, California. The car in the Bronx was attacked by "vandals" within 10 min of its "abandonment." The first to arrive were a family—father, mother, and young son—who removed the radiator and battery. Within 24 h, virtually everything of value had been removed. Then random destruction began—windows were smashed, parts torn off, upholstery ripped. The car in Palo Alto sat untouched for more than a week. Then Zimbardo smashed part of it with a sledgehammer. Soon, passers-by were joining in. Sadly, within a few hours, the car had been turned upside down and utterly destroyed.

Graffiti's Influence on Other Behaviors

Recently, the Broken Windows theory has been further supported by new research conducted by behavioral scientists Keizer et al. (2008). These researchers ran a number of fascinating field experiments to test whether subtle signs of disorder in the environment could create bad behavior in other domains. In one experiment, Keizer and his colleagues found the perfect setting for their test: an alleyway by a shopping mall where shoppers typically parked their bikes. While the shoppers were at the mall, the researchers affixed a store's advertisement on the handlebar of each bicycle with an elastic band. The researchers then either (A) left the alleyway alone just as they found it or (B) added graffiti to it. Because there were no garbage bins in the area, the shoppers who returned from the mall either had to take the advertisement with them or litter it. Which study group (A or B) do you think littered more often?

The results revealed that for study group A, 33 % of the bicycle owners littered the paper affixed to the handlebar on the ground when there was no graffiti present. Amazingly, when the local environment was vandalized with graffiti, the number of bicycle owners who littered increased to a whopping 69 %.

What Does This Mean to Food Safety?

The implications of this research for food safety are clear. The findings demonstrate how powerful subtle cues in someone's environment or work location can be in terms of influencing people's behavior. This research suggests that, as leaders, we should be very careful about the conditions that we tolerate related to disorder, disrepair, and a lack of cleanliness in food manufacturing facilities, food service, and retail food establishments.

Although they may not seem critically important, visible signs of norm violations such as disorder, disrepair, and a lack of cleanliness might normalize elicit undesired behaviors as the norm in other and even more important compliance areas of food safety. As a food safety professional, tolerating or choosing to not respond to a dirty floor, a cluttered shelving unit, or a missing floor or ceiling tile, could be more important than you think.

What broken windows are you tolerating? And what should you do to address and prevent them?

Chapter 8
Learning from the Right Way or Wrong Way?

If you were to board a trans-Atlantic flight knowing you would encounter difficult or extreme weather conditions along the way, who would you prefer to be in the cockpit of the plane? A group of rookie pilots who just graduated from flight school or a captain with a team that had thousands of hours of flying time under their belts, under a wide range of difficult conditions?

Similarly, imagine having to undergo a serious but rare surgery. Who would you want to perform it, the recent graduate from the local medical school or a specialist in a bigger city who has performed that same, rare surgery over a 100 times?

The answers to these questions are obvious. In fact, they are so obvious that they are no-brainers, but why is that? Its because we all know that to be an expert – a real expert that rarely makes errors – receiving training is not enough. Experience matters. And in some professions, where an error can result in life or death, experience matters even more.

Now, do not get me wrong. I realize a pilot's error that causes an airliner to crash is not equivalent to the many errors retail employees may commit. However, there is an important point to be made here, especially as it relates to food safety, where we should all strive for excellence 100 % of the time.

Why Experience Matters

Experience teaches us things that training alone, as generally conducted, cannot. When we actually have to do something many times over, its different than just hearing about it in the classroom or on a computer-based module. We get to experience firsthand what works, what does not work, and what we need to do to optimize our performance. In the book, *How We Decide*, author John Lehrer states, *"Expertise is simply the wisdom that emerges from cellular error."* In other words, we are all human and all systems are not full-proof, so, as much as we hate them, errors

© Springer Science+Business Media New York 2015
F. Yiannas, *Food Safety = Behavior*, Food Microbiology and Food Safety,
DOI 10.1007/978-1-4939-2489-9_8

happen. Therefore, errors – as much as we should strive to prevent them – should not simply be discouraged, punished, or ridiculed. They MUST be learned from, as they are a common route to true expertise and, more importantly, prevention.

The Science of Training: What Really Works?

Organizations worldwide spend billions of dollars annually training their employees in hopes of imparting knowledge, skills, and behavior change. These organizations believe that training their employees will help them (among other things) compete, be safe and compliant, provide better service, and reduce errors. But is all training effective? Of course not. And is there any evidence that all this training is working? I think we can all relate to training we have attended that was voluminous, non-applicable, ineffective, boring, and dull.

But what if I told you that there is a growing field of science demonstrating that there is a better way to train? A method of training that simultaneously imparts knowledge, skills, and, most importantly, 'experience.' Better yet, we can let employees gain years of valuable experience without letting them make the more critical mistakes on the job that might cause serious consequences or harm. Would you be interested?

What Training Firefighters Can Teach Us

Joung et al. (2006), three behavioral researchers in Australia, wanted to know just that. These researchers wanted to test whether they could create a series of training sessions where students would not have to make errors themselves, but instead could learn from other peoples' mistakes–actual or potential. Some of these mistakes would be selected and presented by trainers as good illustrations from which to gain experience and learn.

Joung et al., tested this hypothesis on enrollees in an instructional program for firefighters. In their training sessions, all students were presented with case studies that exposed trainees to the past choices of other firefighters (i.e. firefighting stories based on real incidents). However, as part of the research, the class was randomly divided into two groups.

In Group One, the trainees received scenarios that contained errors made by firefighters (underestimation of resource requirements, miscalculation of changing weather conditions, etc.), many of which resulted in tragic consequences. In Group Two, the trainees received similar real-life scenarios, except this time the case studies were presented without errors (i.e., success stories). For this group, the instructors focused on the successful choices made by the firefighters (i.e. how they did things the right way).

After these initial training sessions, given through real-world, case studies (one emphasizing the errors and consequences; and the other emphasizing successful, right choices), the two groups were presented with a set of new scenarios for problem solving and skill demonstration. In this part of the experiment, both groups One and Two were presented with identical sets of scenarios. Remember, the only difference between the two groups was their training. Which group do you think performed better?

As you might expect, participants in Group One (training that emphasized errors and consequences) outperformed Group Two (training that emphasized success stories) in identifying problems in the firefighting practices. In post-training evaluations, those who received the error-based training scored significantly better on subsequent tests of their judgment and adaptive thinking in firefighting situations.

What Does This Mean to Food Safety?

The implications of this research for food safety are clear. When teaching food safety to employees, its important to teach them what right looks like, such as the right temperatures to cook or maintain food as required by law. They should also be able to identify foods defined as potentially hazardous, the common pathogens associated with these foods, and what to do to inactivate them and prevent cross-contamination.

However, Joung et al.'s (2006) research also suggests that we need to do more in our training. We should also provide trainees with experience by using real-world case studies of prior outbreaks documented in society, the errors committed that failed to prevent these outbreaks, and the consequences experienced by real people (illnesses and deaths). Thereafter, new life-like scenarios should be presented to test knowledge, prevention judgment, and adaptive thinking.

Think about this lesson and the food safety training you are currently conducting. Are you simply imparting knowledge, or are you influencing behavior and providing experience too?

In closing, remember that food safety requires teaching others how to do things the right way. However, counter-intuitively, teaching them the right way might be more impactful by also illustrating the wrong way.

Chapter 9
Make Food Safety the Social Norm

In this chapter, I want to share some thoughts on a behavioral science principle called *"social norm"*–since it directly relates to creating a food safety culture, enhancing employee compliance, and, in general, group behavior.

According to BusinessDictionary.com, social norm is defined as a *"pattern of behavior in a particular group, community, or culture, accepted as normal and to which an individual is expected to conform."* Bestselling author and psychologist Robert Cialdini states, *"People are more willing to take a recommended action if they see evidence that many others, especially similar others, are taking it."*

Believe it or not, most humans are social beings. We depend on others and want to be liked by others. Additionally, we want to fit in with certain social groups (our circle of friends, workgroup, or local community). Although this desire is not the same for everyone, as you can always find the occasional maverick who wants to stand-out, it is generally true for most people, and clear behavioral science evidence supports this principle. More importantly, there are clear societal benefits to the principle of social norms.

Pointing and Gawking Experiment

As a very basic example of this principle, many of you have probably heard of the *Pointing and Gawking Experiment* by Milgram et al. (1969) in a General Psychology course. This experiment by Milgram determined that if a single person stands on a street corner and looks up, about 40 % of the individuals that walk by will do the same. Many people walking by will simply not pay attention to solely one person looking up. However, what do you think happens when you place multiple people on that same street corner looking up? Yes, that's right.

© Springer Science+Business Media New York 2015
F. Yiannas, *Food Safety = Behavior*, Food Microbiology and Food Safety,
DOI 10.1007/978-1-4939-2489-9_9

As people walk by, a large majority of those walking by (almost 85 %) look up as well. Before you know it, there is a large group of people standing on that same street corner looking up at nothing!

Solomon Asche Experiment

If that experiment does not convince you, here is a more persuasive experiment about a person's willingness to conform just to fit into a social group. It's called the *Solomon Asche Experiment*. In this study by Asche (1951), a group of individuals were placed in a class room with one person being a sole, unknown experimental subject. All other individuals (students) in the room were part of the experiment. Individuals in the room were asked by an instructor (who was also in on the experiment) to choose which of the three lines on the right side of a board matched the length of a line on the left side of the board. The task was repeated several times. On some occasions, the other "test subjects" intentionally and unanimously choose a wrong length line. Imagine yourself in this situation. If you were the sole, unknown experimental subject in the room, what would you do? Would you go along with the majority opinion (obviously being able to see clearly that it was the wrong length), or would you trust your own eyes and go with your own correct answer?

As amazing as it may sound, in Solomon's experiment, about one third of the test subjects who were placed in this situation went along with the rest of the group, the clearly erroneous majority.

I could go on and on with examples, but I will not. The bottom line is that many people will do what other people do – just to fit in. It's a proven fact of human behavior.

Well Intentioned, Poorly Communicated

Every year, during National Clean Hands Week in the U.S., its common to see headlines in the news emphasizing that a large percentage of people do not wash their hands after using the restroom. As an example, here is an actual headline from one major news outlet that read, "Restroom Study Finds Hand Washing on the Decline." The news article was reported following a study conducted by the American Society for Microbiology in which researchers observed the behavior of almost 6,100 adults at six locations in four major cities in the U.S. (Atlanta, Chicago, New York, and San Francisco). In the study, they found that approximately 1 out of every 4 people did not wash their hands after using the restroom in a public setting. Most of the news articles following the study emphasized that many people did not wash their hands, as illustrated by the headline above. However, while their motives were probably focused on attracting readers, these headlines reveal a real lack of understanding of human behavior and the principle of social norm. As opposed to emphasizing the minority that did not wash their hands, their stories would have been more beneficial if they emphasized how many actually did wash their hands, thereby, communicating that a majority of people actually do wash their hands after using the restroom. In this manner, those that do not wash might feel social pressure to fit in and start washing!

Making Hand Washing the Social Norm

Lapinski et al. (2013) wanted to know if this premise was correct. In other words, does how you communicate whether or not people wash their hands actually influence the desired behavior? In their study of college-aged men conducted at Michigan State University (MSU), males were surveyed and self-reported washing their hands 75 % of the time (similar to the percentage often observed in observational studies documented in the literature.) To test their hypotheses, signs were posted in restrooms on the University's campus that read, "*4 out of 5 Males Wash Their Hands.*" The signs also contained pictures of students wearing MSU hats; thereby emphasizing that hand washing was the social norm on campus. The researchers then stationed themselves, inconspicuously, in the restrooms and actually recorded the frequency of hand-washing behavior. Of interest, 86 % of the men observed in experimentally signed restrooms actually washed their hands. The researchers reported that men exposed to a primed message that conveys hand washing as the social norm were more likely to wash their hands (and run the water longer!) than participants not exposed to the messages.

What Does This Mean to Food Safety?

The implications from these studies are real and impactful. Many individuals are moved to act or comply with certain behaviors just because they see other people behaving in the same way. Therefore, part of your job as a food safety professional involves taking tactical and intentional actions that help others see that food safety is the social norm and part of your organization's culture.

In addition to the hand-washing example cited in the study above, how can you accomplish this goal? What about communicating the large number of establishments that pass inspections, rather than emphasizing the smaller percentage that fail? While I could go on and on with real-world examples, I am sure you can come up with more on your own.

In closing, think about the way you communicate food safety compliance or a lack of compliance. Do you communicate in such a way that influences others to want to be in compliance and part of the social norm? Remember, to be successful in advancing food safety, you will need to go beyond the fundamentals of food science and apply principles of behavioral science as well.

Make food safety the Social Norm. You won't be successful without doing so.

Chapter 10
Shining a Light on Food Safety

How important is the effect of lighting on food safety? On almost every food safety inspection conducted around the world, whether it's at a retail establishment, a food service location, or in a food manufacturing facility, there is a question requiring the auditor to check on the facility's lighting. But what if I told you the reason the food inspector checks the lighting might just be for the wrong reason, would you believe me?

Why is lighting so often examined by food safety auditors today? Generally, they check lighting for one of two reasons. First, the inspector is required to examine the lighting to ensure that any bulbs or glass lamps used in the facility or on equipment are shatter-proof or protected in a manner that prevents broken glass from making its way into food. Second, inspectors check the lighting of an establishment to ensure that adequate illumination exists for sanitary reasons. Adequate levels of illumination allow operators and regulators to more easily observe if the establishment's conditions are soiled, dirty, or require cleaning. In fact, the Food Code goes as far as to outline in detail specific lighting intensity requirements. For example, walk-in refrigeration units and dry food storage areas must provide at least 110 lux (10 ft. candles) at a distance of 75 cm (30 in.) above the floor. Wherever packaged foods are sold and inside equipment such as reach-in and under-counter refrigerators, the Food Code states the light intensity must be at least 220 lux (20 fc).

However, as per my opening question, what if I told you lighting might influence much more. Previous research has demonstrated lighting's effect on crime. Researchers have concluded that more lighting discourages crime by increasing the likelihood of witnesses seeing the crime.

But what about lighting's effects on other behaviors not involving crime? Does lighting make a difference? Zhong et al. (2010) wanted an answer to that question. They sought to investigate whether or not lighting conditions would affect people's honesty within organizations.

© Springer Science+Business Media New York 2015
F. Yiannas, *Food Safety = Behavior*, Food Microbiology and Food Safety,
DOI 10.1007/978-1-4939-2489-9_10

The Difference Eight Light Bulbs Can Make

In their first experiment, they had participants work in either a well-lit room or in a room with three quarters of the lights not working properly. They asked participants to complete a 20 problem math quiz under time constraints, and told the participants that they would get compensated for each correct answer. At the end of the 5 min quiz, the participants were told to score their own work on a reporting sheet and turn it in to collect their newly earned cash. Unknown to the participants, the researchers had a way to link participants' work sheets to their reporting sheets, which they turned in for payment. In this way, the researchers were able to measure the difference between the actual number of correct answers and the number of correct answers reported by the participants.

Participants in both rooms had the same number of actual correct answers, but 61 % of those in the dimly lit room cheated on their self-reported answers while only 24 % in the well-lit room cheated! This supports the idea that darkness increases dishonest behavior. Thought about a little differently, by simply better illuminating the room where the study took place with 8 fluorescent light bulbs, dishonesty was reduced by an amazing 37 %!

In another set of experiments, researchers wanted to know whether lighting itself or simply the perception of lighting could influence behavior. To research this question, participants were invited to "test" a new pair of glasses (either sunglasses or clear glasses). After donning the glasses, participants were asked to interact with an anonymous stranger via a computer based game where they could split $6 between themselves and the anonymous participant (which was actually the investigator in another room, but the participants didn't know that). Participants who wore the sunglasses gave on average $0.90 less (14 % less) than those who wore the clear glasses. Moreover, participants who wore sunglasses reported feeling more anonymous than those wearing clear glasses. The researchers' statistical analyses of the results revealed that the feeling of anonymity accounted for the difference in giving between participants who wore the sunglasses versus the clear glasses.

In summary, the researchers concluded that the feeling of anonymity created by a dimly lit room or by wearing sunglasses led to increased dishonesty. They use the term 'disinhibit' to describe this phenomenon.

What Does This Mean to Food Safety?

The implications from this research are important and extremely relevant to food safety. The results of this and other studies suggest that darkness increases a person's feeling of anonymity and thus can "disinhibit" dishonest behaviors. While your initial focus from reading this study might be on lighting alone, it should not be. Instead, you should focus more broadly on conditions that promote anonymity (including lighting). The research is clear. When people feel that they can operate "anonymously," they are more likely to behave in dishonest and unethical ways.

Increased anonymity equals reduced accountability. From a food safety perspective, feelings of increased anonymity among employees are likely to lead to feelings of reduced accountability and, thereby, to an increase in non-compliant behaviors. Conversely, Carver and Scheier (1998) have shown that increased lighting or anything else that results in increased self-awareness (cameras, mirrors, etc.) results in a more reflective self-regulation of desired behaviors.

Think about these findings and what they might mean to food safety. For example:

- Could we enhance desired food safety behaviors in employees and minimize the feeling of anonymity by simply better illuminating workplaces through additional fixtures and smarter building designs (windows, open work areas, etc.)?
- What else can we do to decrease feelings of anonymity in the workplace? While I can tell you from experience that large, open kitchens exposed to the customers' view put pressure on employees to keep the kitchen cleaner, I cannot help but think: does it also increase compliance with desired hand washing and hygiene behaviors by the employees who work in that kitchen?
- Finally, what does this principle mean for food suppliers? If suppliers think that they will be caught shorting you an ounce of product in each bag by substituting an inferior, less expensive ingredient, do you think they will try shorting you? Of course not.

In closing, while retail establishments pay a considerable amount of attention to lighting's effect on mood in customer service areas, fitting rooms, and on product showroom displays, its often an oversight or an afterthought in back-room employee areas.

Remember: look for ways to shine a light on food safety – both figuratively and literally. It's more important than you think.

Chapter 11
What Nouns, Verbs, & Voting Can Teach Us About Food Safety

If you are like me, the never-ending political cycle, ensures that you receive your fair share of political emails, phone calls, and advertisements. While it may seem a bit overwhelming, of particular interest to this study is that much of the strategies being used in political campaigns these days are actually founded in behavioral science principles. Therefore, I thought I would share a basic question often asked by political strategists–*how do you get people to vote?* The answer to this question is not only interesting, but it could help you enhance your organization's performance in food safety.

Enhancing Voter Turnout

Getting people to vote – otherwise known as voter turnout–is critical to winning an election. One simple and effortless method that works in getting voters to the polls can be discerned from a behavioral study conducted by researchers at Stanford and Harvard (Bryan et al. 2011). In this study, researchers randomly sampled registered voters in the state of California prior to the 2008 elections and divided them into two separate groups (A & B). They then contacted the study participants and asked them to complete similar, yet subtly different surveys.

In the first group (A), participants were asked to complete a series of short questions that referred to them (the survey participants) by using a self-relevant noun: *voter*. The critical research question read like this–*How important is it for you to be a voter in the upcoming election?*

In the second group (B), the questions were nearly identical, but they referred to voting as a behavior by using the word *vote* (a verb). This time the research question read–*How important is it for you to vote in the upcoming election?*

© Springer Science+Business Media New York 2015
F. Yiannas, *Food Safety = Behavior*, Food Microbiology and Food Safety,
DOI 10.1007/978-1-4939-2489-9_11

After the election, the researchers used official state records to determine which survey participants had actually voted and which ones had not voted. Of the two groups, which one do you think had the greater turnout?

Of interest, the researchers found that using a noun (voter) vs. a verb (vote) in the pre-election questionnaire had a significant effect on voter turnout. Participants in the noun-conditioned group (A) voted at a significantly higher rate (90 %) than those in the verb-conditioned group (B – 79 %). In fact, the researchers concluded that merely framing the act of voting a little differently by labeling participants prior to the election as *voters*, as opposed to merely focusing on their behavior, *voting*, they were able to increase voter turnout by an impressive 11 %.

Think about the significance of these findings. Politicians often go to great lengths and spend huge sums of money trying to get people to vote. However, as this research reveals, something as small as framing how people perceive themselves, as opposed to their behavior, actually achieved better results.

What Does This Mean to Food Safety?

The implications of this research are clear. Subtle and almost effortless changes in phrasing, such as talking about food safety or compliance using nouns (culturally desirable traits)–instead of verbs (behaviors)–may have a significant and positive effect on influencing others and enhancing their compliance with your requests.

Why is this the case? According to researchers, labeling others with desirable self-expressions helps them see themselves as being part of a favorable social group (people who vote are viewed more favorably by society than those who do not vote). Thus, you are enhancing a person's likelihood to take actions to live up to that view, request, or expectation of them.

Think about these findings and how you might use nouns instead of verbs to further strengthen the food safety performance of your organization.

For example, consider a health education outreach program trying to teach parents in a community about how to protect their families from foodborne illness. Instead of focusing on the desired behavior (the verb) needed to take place, frame the conversation around a parent's role as protector of their family's wellbeing – and then emphasize the desired food safety behavior. The research suggests that this approach might just be more effective.

In summary, remember that referring to others using socially desirable terms (such as Food Safety Partners or Food Safety Culture Keepers) prior to explaining the desired behavior you are asking them to perform – rather than merely requesting that they adhere to the behavior alone–is likely to yield enhanced compliance and better results.

Chapter 12
Birds of a Feather Might Influence Food Safety for Better

I am sure you have heard of the age-old adage, *"birds of a feather flock together."* You may have even used the phrase yourself. But what does this adage have to do with food safety? Maybe more than you think.

In nature, birds of a single species actually do flock together. It's a fact. Ornithologists explain this grouping as a pro-social behavior amongst a flock of birds, because there is safety in numbers that reduces their risk of being attacked by predators.

However, when related to human behavior, the adage *"birds of a feather flock together"* is something often said to imply that people who have similar characteristics or interests will often choose to spend time together.

This adage is reported to have gained common popularity after being used in literature during the mid sixteenth century. However, some believe the phrase actually originates from ancient Greece. In Aristotle's *Rhetoric*, he notes that people *"love those who are like themselves."*

Homophily

In the 1950s, sociologist coined the term "homophily" to explain the tendency of human beings to associate or bond with others similar to themselves. Since that time, McPherson et al. (2001) have concluded that more than 100 studies have demonstrated that homophily in some form breeds connection. People look to connect with people of similar race, ethnicity, age, gender, education, occupational roles, social class, and more.

At first, sociologist believed that homophily might limit a person's social world by narrowing the diversity of information they receive and the attitudes they might

© Springer Science+Business Media New York 2015   41
F. Yiannas, *Food Safety = Behavior*, Food Microbiology and Food Safety,
DOI 10.1007/978-1-4939-2489-9_12

form. However, more recently, the concept of homophily has been viewed as a potentiality beneficial and strategic concept to use when attempting to influence people's attitudes, views, and behaviors.

Principle of Likeness

In his classic book, *Influence: The Psychology of Persuasion,* Dr. Robert Cialdini (1993), states that we tend to like people similar to us, whether its based on personality, background, life-style, or occupation. He describes how similarity can to be used to increase compliance. As an amazing illustration of this point, in 1963, researcher F. B. Evans used demographic data from insurance company records to demonstrate that prospects were more likely to purchase a policy from a salesperson that was akin to them in age, religion, politics, or even cigarette-smoking habits.

Additionally, McPherson et al. (2001) describe how people who are more structurally similar to one another are much more likely to have interpersonal communication on specific issues, and how they are more likely to pay attention to one another's positions. As a result, these similarities lead them to have greater influence over one another.

It is also well documented that people who occupy similar positions within a workplace or profession often influence each other. Employees are very likely to have ties to others who occupy the same jobs.

Likeness and Adoption of Health-Related Behaviors

As we have seen, people are more likely to be influenced by others who are similar to themselves. But can this principle be used to promote adoption of desired health-related behaviors? One researcher at the Massachusetts Institute of Technology (MIT) wanted to know just that.

Centola (2011) defined a study to measure if a health-related behavior could be influenced through homophily. To test his hypothesis, he recruited 710 participants through an internet-based social network. Participants arriving for the study were randomly divided into one of two experimental conditions – a homophilous (similar) population condition and an unstructured population condition. The two groups were then further subdivided into what was called network neighborhoods of about 72 participants.

The study involved measuring whether individuals made a decision to adopt an internet-based diet diary. The network was open for all to see and included information about each participant, such as level of fitness, amount of exercise, body mass index, etc. A seed person in each network neighborhood initiated the study by adopting the diet diary. Once they did, all others in the network would receive a notification that one of their buddies had started using the diary and they could then decide to start using it too.

Amazingly, the researchers concluded that homophily (similarity to others) significantly increased the likelihood that study participants would adopt the desired healthy behavior, in this case using the internet-diet diary.

What Does This Mean to Food Safety?

The inferences from this research are clear. Similarity breeds connection and connection leads to greater influence over another person's thoughts, attitudes, and behaviors. Thus, similarity can be used to enhance compliance with desired behaviors, especially in the workplace.

How might this fundamental principle about human nature be used to enhance food safety? Let's consider a few options.

- Instead of asking the Chief Executive Officer or the Vice President of Food Safety to narrate a training video for front-line employees about the importance of food safety, research suggests that we might be more effective by having the message delivered by an employee within the workplace that is familiar to their colleagues and occupies a similar position within the company instead.
- In a global company, it is not uncommon to have a person from Headquarters deliver food safety messages that are often relayed to front-line employees in various markets. Usually, this spokesperson has very little in common to the intended audience due to differences in nationality, language, or occupational role. While this approach may be appropriate at times, the research suggests that using this strategy too often, without considering the importance of homophily, may backfire or simply have no effect at all.

Think about these findings and what they might mean to enhancing food safety within your business.

In closing, remember that birds of a feather flock together. And they might just be more effective at influencing food safety for better as well.

Chapter 13
Keep Food Safety in Mind by Making It Rhyme

When communicating an important concept or thought, whether it is in the spoken or written form, good communicators strive to do it in a manner that is memorable. Strategies to make communication more memorable include linking it to something visual, using repetition, and storytelling.

Age-Old Tradition

Today there are numerous methods that can be used to try to get people to remember things. Before the widespread use of print, oral traditions depended much more heavily on human memory for the preservation of information. Therefore, in preliterate eras, communication had to appeal to one's ear to make it memorable, or else it might be forgotten.

One clever method our ancestors used to make communication more memorable was through the use of aphorisms. You might be asking yourself, what in the world is an aphorism?

Webster's dictionary defines an aphorism as *a short phrase that expresses a true and wise idea*. Researchers believe the first recorded use of the term was in the *Aphorisms of Hippocrates*. In modern times, aphorisms are generally understood to be concise statements containing a truth or observation cleverly and succinctly written (or stated). You can think of them as a proverb, which often rhymes.

Rhyming Helps Us Remember

Studies have repeatedly shown that rhymes can help us remember ideas. They help concepts stick with us over time. In fact, rhymes are so simple and effective that they are often used to help very young children learn how to talk and read. Think of

© Springer Science+Business Media New York 2015
F. Yiannas, *Food Safety = Behavior*, Food Microbiology and Food Safety,
DOI 10.1007/978-1-4939-2489-9_13

Dr Seuss's famous children books like *Cat in the Hat* or *Hop on Pop*. According to Kornei Chukovsky, famous author of Russian children's books, *"There is hardly a child whose verbal development in this early period does not use linking pairs – most often rhythmic pairs – of sounds and words."*

The effect of rhyming on helping us remember things has to do with something called mnemonics. The term "mnemonic" is derived from the Greek root word for memory. Its basically a method or tool used to help us remember things. A variety of popular mnemonic methods exist, ranging from the method of loci (a technique in which you associate the new with the familiar) to acronyms (using the first letter of each word in a phrase) to rhymes.

However, rhymes are considered one of the easiest ways to enhance memory and recollection. By rhyming information, our brains can encode it more easily through something neurologists refer to as "acoustic encoding." Bottom line, rhymes clearly enhance memory and recollection.

Poetic Effect on Believability

Rhyme and rhythm are already well proven mnemonic techniques to help in aiding memory, but can they enhance believability? Two researchers, McGlone and Tofighbakhsh (2000), at Lafayette College wanted to look at this premise in more detail. They wanted to know whether aphorisms, proverbs that rhyme, influenced people's perception of their accuracy about human behavior. In others words, they wanted to see if aphorisms enhanced believability.

To do this, the researchers recruited 120 undergraduate students as participants in a study, all native English speakers. The researchers then developed a list of 30 pairs of matching aphorism or proverbs. One saying in each pair was rephrased to communicate the exact same message, except in this case it did not rhyme.

The students were then divided into two groups and asked to read the 30 sayings. One group of participants received sayings that rhymed. For example, this group read sayings such as *"woes unite foes"* or *"life is mostly strife."*

The other group of participants received the same proverbs, but their proverbs were rephrased so as not to rhyme. For example, this group received sayings that read, *"woes unite enemies"* or *"life is mostly struggle."*

Participants were instructed to read each aphorism and to rate it on a scale from 1 (not at all accurate) to 9 (very accurate) on whether they thought it was an accurate description of human behavior.

Which version do you think participants said was more accurate, the rhyming or non-rhyming version? Yes, you got it. Participants rated the rhyming sayings to be more believable, even though they claimed that whether the proverb rhymed or not had no influence on their determination of the phrase's believability.

Why were the rhyming versions of the sayings perceived to be more believable? The researchers suggest that it is probably due to something referred to as *"process-ing fluency."* Processing fluency refers to the ease at which information is processed in a person's brain. It is believed that the easier it is to process information, the more credible the message will be and the more likely it is to influence someone to action.

What Does This Mean to Food Safety?

The findings from this research are interesting. It suggests that when communicating important truths that we want people to believe, understand, take action on, and remember, how we do it matters. Rather than trying to reach front-line employees and consumers with long-winded sentences about food safety written by scientists, regulators, and academics, maybe we should employ the methods of Hippocrates and use short, rhyming phrases.

I cannot help but think about the important contributing factors of foodborne disease (cooking, cooling, refrigeration, hand washing, etc.) and whether or not a rhyming, succinct statement of proper behaviors regarding these concepts would do more to make the message memorable and actionable than merely listing facts and procedures.

In closing, remember to "*practice food safety each day to prevent foodborne illness*" or should I say, "*practice food safety each day to keep foodborne illness at bay.*"

Chapter 14
Making Scents of Food Safety

Have you ever paused to consider how different smells, odors, and aromas affect us? If you are like most people, the smell of garbage, sewage, or rotten fruit can elicit a pretty strong response of disgust. On the other hand, most people enjoy the smell of freshly baked bread, floral scents, and spring rain. Think about these scents and the emotions they conjure. How do they make you feel?

Interestingly enough, previous research has demonstrated that scents can do more than just affect our senses. They also can influence our behaviors, both positively and negatively.

Willingness to Help Others

Some researchers have documented that smells can actually increase our willingness to help others. Guéguen (2012), advancing this line of research, looked at the effects of a pleasant scent on the spontaneous actions of helping others.

Guéguen tested his hypothesis in a shopping mall, and chose locations based on their aromas: either in front of a clothing store or in front of a store with pleasant food smells, such as bakery. An experimenter would stand near the store window and appear as if he or she was looking inside the store. After selecting a subject from someone passing by, the experimenter would walk in front of the shopper, rummage through a handbag, and intentionally drop a glove without appearing to notice the accident. Discrete observers would note the shopper's gender, approximate age, and whether or not they notified the experimenter that they had dropped something.

Two hundred test subjects were used in each test area. Seventy-seven percent of the people in the pleasant smelling area helped the experimenter by alerting them to the dropped item. In contrast, only 52.5 % of people in the unscented area helped the experimenter. The researchers concluded that this difference was significant. In

© Springer Science+Business Media New York 2015   49
F. Yiannas, *Food Safety = Behavior*, Food Microbiology and Food Safety,
DOI 10.1007/978-1-4939-2489-9_14

other words, the shoppers that smelled pleasant odors, unknowingly, were more likely to engage in helping behavior.

Aromas and Safe Driving

Even more support exists in the literature for pleasant fragrances improving desired behaviors, including safety related behaviors. In an intriguing series of experiments, Baron and Kalsher (1998) measured how pleasant aromas and gifts impacted a participant's simulated driving performance. Psychology students volunteered for the study in which they used a joystick to control a car in a computer simulation. Throughout the study's course, they had to keep the car pointed at a distant object just as drivers have to keep their cars centered in driving lanes. Warning signs would intermittently appear, and the participants had to respond while maintaining steady steering. The experimenters used the gift condition as a control, which actually decreased performance. However, a pleasant lemon scent from an air freshener increased cognitive ability and driver performance, which ultimately improved safety.

Baron and Kalsher speculate that this effect could be due to increased alertness. Based on their findings, they suggest that drivers could be monitored for drowsiness and alerted by spraying scents into the air whenever drowsiness is detected. They also mention that drivers could have the option to voluntarily spray the scents when they feel tired.

Taken together, these research findings support the idea that aroma can affect human behavior, both in terms of helpfulness and safety. In what other ways do you think aromas might influence behavior?

What Does This Mean to Food Safety?

These studies' results are interesting. In an environment with pleasant scents, people were significantly more likely to help others than in an aroma neutral environment. Moreover, pleasant aromas improved safety-related tasks and performance. Pause for a moment to think about this. A subtle, environmental cue, such as an aroma, can have a powerful and unconscious influence on human behavior.

While aromas, both good and bad, are quite common in food and agricultural settings, their influence on human behaviors is seldom considered. However, these findings suggest that aromas could have some very important implications for food safety and our profession.

First, in what situations could we intentionally scent the environment with a pleasant smell that could positively influence desired behaviors? "Helping" behaviors could include anything from going the extra mile for a customer to picking up some slack for someone whose department is slammed. Most food safety behaviors, such as hand washing and glove use, fall into the category of pro-social or caring actions, which could also be influenced. Also, scents that improve cognitive ability could help employees follow more complex food safety procedures.

Second, what about those smells present in the industry that are not particularly pleasant? Generally, offensive odors are abated, especially if they can be smelled by customers. However, could offensive odors in non-customer areas, if unabated, unintentionally dissuade employees from being helpful or behaving in desired ways? Many of the scents come from chemicals or processes that are vital to the operation, but if an approximately 25 % difference in behavior is what is at stake, what can you do to minimize or improve the smells?

In closing, think about how you might use these findings and investigate how they might improve food safety. While we all know that food safety makes sense, it might be scents that help improve food safety.

Chapter 15
Font Style & Food Safety

As the legendary basketball coach John Wooden once said, *"It's the little details that are vital. Little things make bigger things happen."* With this thought in mind, I would like to ask you to think about something you have probably never paid much attention to because you might have viewed it as insignificant or as a simple matter of preference.

Could the font style you use to communicate food safety information, whether it's Times New Roman, Papyrus, Richard, **Arial**, *Freestyle Script*, or any other font you like to use, influence whether people understand your message and remember it?

While some of the flowery fonts that people like to use, like *Freestyle*, might frustrate you and be a little more difficult to read, does this concept of font-choice really matter for the more typical scripts used in the business world today, such as **Ariel**?

Several behavioral psychologist, Gasser et al. (2005) wanted to know just that. In particular, they wanted to research whether the presence of serifs on a font and how the font was spaced affected reading comprehension. A serif is the little mark on the bottom of letters which make the letters seem like they are sitting on a line. Times New Roman, which is the font style used in this book, has serifs. Look at this "f"; do you see the little 'wings' or 'flanges' on the bottom which make it look like it's sitting on a line? That's a serif. This "f," lacking the little 'wings,' is called sans-serif or without-serif. Additionally, fonts either have a uniform spacing between letters or the spacing differs depending on the size of the letter.

In the study conducted by Gasser et al., 149 research participants, all undergraduate psychology students, were randomly divided into four groups. Each group was given a one page, single-spaced memo from a local health clinic on tuberculosis, which was printed in one of four font styles (Courier, Palatino, Helvetica, or Monaco). Courier represented a mono-spaced serif. Palatino represented a proportionally spaced serif. Helvetica represented a proportional san serif, and Monaco represented a mono-spaced san serif.

In the research exercise, participants were given as much time as needed to read the memo, although most completed reading it within 8 min. Afterwards, they were

© Springer Science+Business Media New York 2015
F. Yiannas, *Food Safety = Behavior*, Food Microbiology and Food Safety,
DOI 10.1007/978-1-4939-2489-9_15

given a series of unrelated questions, which were intentionally planned as a distrac-
tive task. In order to test their knowledge and retention of information regarding
tuberculosis, each participant was asked six open-ended questions about the important portions of the memo they had read on tuberculosis.

Analysis of the study results revealed that letter spacing did not have a significant
effect on the ability of participants to recall or remember the information they had
read. However, participants who read the memos in serif fonts (Courier and Palatino)
had a significantly higher ability (9 %) to recall and remember critical or important
portions of information in the memo they had read than those who read the memos
in san serif.

Why is that? The researchers theorize that the presence of serifs increases the
perception that text progresses on a line. Therefore, the reader can put less effort
into reading the text and more effort into understanding it. In other words, they
concluded that ease of reading is likely to result in enhanced understanding and
memory retention.

Ease of Readability Matters

Numerous studies have previously shown that even small increases in readability
matters. For example, Murphy (1947) demonstrated that he could increase the readability of an article from 43 % to 60 % by simply reducing the level of difficulty
required to read it from a 9th grade reading level to a 6th grade level.

Other studies have also shown that ease of reading can be used to predict how
much of an article is actually read, which is referred to as reading depth, persistence,
or perseverance. In other words, if an article requires too much effort to read or is
too difficult, the reader is unlikely to finish reading it in its entirety and will instead
skim read it.

What Does This Mean to Food Safety?

The findings from this research are clearly of interest. It suggests that by merely being
a little more intentional in font style selection, requiring little effort and no additional
expense, one can significantly improve the likelihood that critical food safety information communicated in writing will be completely read, understood, and retained.

Think about these findings and what they mean to food safety. For example, stop
to consider for a moment all of the communication on food safety that is delivered
in writing. Examples of important food safety instructions and messages that are
communicated in writing include:

• Standard operating procedures
• Food safety checklists

- Laws and regulations
- Training & education curriculums
- Consumer food safety recall messages

Have you ever given a second thought to what font style you were using to communicate these instructions and messages? If you did, it was probably due to personal preference – not because you thought it would be more effective. However, this research suggests that we better stop and think about our selection of font styles in more detail.

Fonts matter. And they could make a significant difference in retention and comprehension.

Chapter 16
Can SOPs Actually Hinder Food Safety?

I would like to begin this chapter with a provocative question; *do written Standard Operation Procedures (SOPs) actually help or hurt food safety?* The simple answer to this question is, it depends.

Over the course of my career, I have worked with numerous compliance professionals who have been, in my view, overly fixated on writing SOPs for food safety in hopes that having well documented procedures would lead to enhanced compliance. Although such initiatives are common and well intentioned, I believe they often miss the mark and, in some instances, do more harm than good. Let me explain.

At the end of the day, what an employee knows about food safety or what is written on a piece of paper – an SOP – is not what is really important. It's what a person does – their behavior – that is key. Remember, you can have the most thoroughly documented food safety practices and SOPs in the world, but if your associates are not putting them into practice, the SOPs are useless.

Now don't get me wrong. I am not against having written procedures. They are necessary and, if done correctly, useful. In fact, as I stated in my book *Food Safety Culture* (2008), many food safety professionals think that the first step in achieving enhanced food safety performance is to make sure all employees have received food safety training. However, while training may be important, achieving success in food safety actually starts much earlier than the training period. It begins by making sure you have created clear, specific, and objective food safety expectations for your associates, and that those expectations are easy to understand and follow. And for some of these expectations, it makes sense for them to be documented.

© Springer Science+Business Media New York 2015
F. Yiannas, *Food Safety = Behavior*, Food Microbiology and Food Safety,
DOI 10.1007/978-1-4939-2489-9_16

If It's Hard to Read, It Must Be Hard to Do

Several behavioral studies have shown that the perceived effort a behavior requires is a good indicator of its likely adoption. Very importantly, studies also demonstrate that the experience of fluency, the ability to read and understand something easily, affects a person's perception of the amount of effort it will take to adopt or perform the desired behavior.

Behavioral psychologists Song and Schwarz (2008) conducted a classic study that proves this point. Song and Schwarz presented research subjects with written exercise instructions. When the instructions were presented in an easy-to-read format and font, the participants assumed that the exercise would take on average 8.2 min to complete. In contrast, when the participants were presented with the same exercise instructions in a difficult format and font, the participants assumed it would take almost twice as long to complete: 15.1 min.

Even more concerning, participants told researchers that when the instructions were presented in the more complicated manner, they assumed that performing the exercise would be more difficult and time consuming. Thus, they were less likely to try incorporating the exercise into their daily routine.

What Does This Mean to Food Safety?

The inferences from this research are clear. If we want employees to adopt or follow a specific food safety behavior, we not only have to design instructions in a simple and easy to use manner, but we also must ensure that the instructions are conceptually clear when we communicate them to our employees (whether verbally or especially in writing).

Therefore, when documenting or writing a work procedure, it is critical that it be written in a clear, visually appealing, and simplified manner. If it's written in a complicated format, the attempt to enhance compliance by having a written SOP in place could actually backfire by making the desired behavior or task seem unduly demanding and overly complex, and, as a result, less likely to be used or followed. Another way to communicate without using longwinded, lengthy, and ineffective SOPs is through the use of visual job aids that depict how the work is to be conducted. Studies have repeatedly shown that visualization facilitates communication and enhances learning.

In summary, remember that in today's fast paced organization, what is not simple is not clear and what is not clear will not get done. So the next time you are writing a food safety procedure, strive for simplicity: do more food safety with fewer words. It could make the difference between success and failure.

Chapter 17
Which One is Better, Written or Verbal?

As a food safety or compliance professional, a common action that you will take during the course of your career will be to ask someone to follow-up on a practice or condition that you have found to be out-of-compliance without being able to go back and observe if the situation has been corrected for yourself. When identifying an issue that needs to be corrected, whether its during an informal tour of a food manufacturing site or a more formally conducted food safety audit, which choice do you think is 'most' effective at getting someone to correct the issue?

(a) A verbal commitment at the time with the person telling you they will fix the issue
(b) A verbal confirmation that the issue has been corrected by calling the person in charge to discuss whether or not it has been done
(c) A verbal confirmation that the issue has been corrected in a face to face meeting with the person in charge, but off-site, so you cannot confirm the correction yourself
(d) Obtaining a written statement from the person summarizing the corrective actions taken to correct the issue through a requested written action plan

Method of Communication and Deception

While all of the methods offered above can work, some are more effective than others. A study conducted by Dr. Jeff Hancock and his colleagues at Cornell University provides some insight into the best answer to this question.

According to a study he designed to evaluate which forms of communication were more likely to contain intentional inaccuracies after making a specific request, he found that 14 % of emails, 27 % of face to face conversations, and 37 % of discussions by phone contained inaccuracies, lies, or stretches of the truth

© Springer Science+Business Media New York 2015
F. Yiannas, *Food Safety = Behavior*, Food Microbiology and Food Safety,
DOI 10.1007/978-1-4939-2489-9_17

According to Toma and Hancock (2012), people are more reluctant to lie in writing because having a permanent record of their communication makes them believe that they are more likely to get caught. This same conclusion is also supported by research conducted by bestselling author and behavioral psychologist, Robert Cialdini (1993), who found that written commitments are more effective at getting people to follow-through on requested actions than verbal commitments.

Why is that? Behavioral psychologists believe that having to write something down on paper tends to work better than a verbal commitment. Verbally, one can more easily stretch the truth or, at a later date, deny statements made, or suggest that they were misunderstood because there is not a formal written record. Think about formal agreements or contracts. There is a reason they are always documented on paper versus simply being verbal commitments.

E-Mail Versus Other Forms of Written Communication

While it's been established that written methods are more effective than verbal ones to ensure people stay true and follow-through on previous commitments, does the form of writing (email, handwritten, etc.) also make a difference?

Three researchers, Naquin et al. (2010), wanted to investigate whether the degree of truthfulness varied depending on the form of written communication used – email versus handwritten. To do so, they conducted a series of studies.

In their first experiment, 48 full-time MBA students were given $89 each and asked to divide it between themselves and another fictional party. The other party did not know the exact amount of money given to the MBA student. They only knew that the dollar amount ranged somewhere between $5 and $100. In the study, there was one pre-condition: the other party had to accept whatever offer was made to them. The MBA students were asked to report the size of the pot and how much the other party would get – using either e-mail or pen and paper.

Students asked to share information via e-mail (versus pen and paper) lied about the amount of money or the size of the pot to be divided 92 % of the time. In contrast, only 64 % of MBA students asked to share this information by pen and paper lied about the size of the pot. While the results of both groups were disturbing, the rate of lying was 'significantly' greater when the students communicated this information by email.

E-mailers also misrepresented the size of the pot as being smaller ($56 dollars), and they felt more justified in awarding the other party just $29 out of the total pot. Students who communicated by pen and paper misrepresented the pot size on average to be $67 and appeared to be a slightly more generous. On average, they shared $34 with the other party.

Naquin, one of the researchers, said, "Keep in mind that both of these media – e-mail and pen-and-paper – are text only. Neither has greater 'communication bandwidth' than the other. Yet we still see a dramatic difference."

In trying to determine if a lack or sense of shared identity contributed to the students' willingness to lie, the researchers set up a second, related experiment with MBA students. As expected, the results of this study indicated that the more familiar students were with the other party, the less deceptive they would be. However, they would still lie regardless of how well they identified with each other, and lying by email was again greater than by pen and paper.

What Does This Mean to Food Safety?

The implications from these research studies are clear. First, if you want to increase the likelihood of a person following-through on a compliance request, ask them to send you their corrective action plan in writing – and do not simply ask them about it by phone or in a meeting. As a result, you will significantly increase the likelihood that it will actually get done.

However, additional research suggests that the method of written communication may matter, whether its handwritten, by email, or by completing something in digital form via a software program or on a computer system.

With the emergence of email and digital online communication tools in the workplace, more research is clearly needed to determine how effective electronic tools are in communicating and documenting the truth.

The implications of these findings on food safety should be further researched. For example, how should corrective actions used to address food safety violations be documented? This research suggests that written confirmation that the corrective action has been taken is likely to be more effective, on average, than a mere verbal confirmation. However, does it matter if the corrective action is documented with pen and paper, email, or digitally in a software program?

Think about these findings and how you might use them for a variety of issues to better enhance follow-through and prevention. For now, until more research is done, know this: if you want to ensure something gets done, ask for it in writing. Studies show that it greatly enhances follow-through and completion.

Chapter 18
Three Degrees of Food Safety

If someone were to ask you what three degrees have to do with food safety, what would your answer be? If you are like most food safety professionals, you will probably think of food temperatures, with three degrees potentially meaning the difference between a food item being fully cooked or undercooked.

Although this answer is true, in this chapter, I want you to think about the concept of three degrees quite differently. Instead of thinking of attributes related to food temperatures, I want to share what three degrees mean in terms of the behavioral sciences and social groups.

If you think about it, in many instances human behavior has more to do with groups than individuals. Ties between people in social groups, like an organization of any significant size, are sometimes more important in influencing the behaviors of others than the words or actions of any single individual. That is because a group of aligned individuals working together can do more than any single person to influence behavior within an organization. And in such instances, the whole of an organization is greater than the sum of its parts.

People Do What Other People Do

The social sciences teach us that there is a tendency for human beings to mimic each other. Behavioral psychologists call this the principle of 'social norm.' In other words, people do what others do. As a classic example, let's review a study conducted by psychologist Morgan Stanley, called the *Pointing and Gawking Experiment*. In this experiment, if a single person stands on a street corner and looks up, about 40 % of the individuals that walk by will do the same. Many people will simply walk by and not pay attention to the single person looking up. However, what do you think happens when you place multiple people on that same street corner looking up? As people walk by, a vast majority (almost 85 %) will look up

© Springer Science+Business Media New York 2015
F. Yiannas, *Food Safety = Behavior*, Food Microbiology and Food Safety,
DOI 10.1007/978-1-4939-2489-9_18

too. And before you know it, there is a large group of people standing on that same street corner looking up – at nothing! Why is it that? At its most basic root, its because people do what other people do.

Three Degrees of Influence

Even more interesting, recent studies demonstrate that our social influence can go much further than simply affecting the people we know or come into direct contact with. According to studies published by Nicholas Christakis and James Fowler in their book, *Connected, The Surprising Power of Our Social Networks and How They Shape Our Lives*, the spread of influence in social networks tends to obey what they call the "Three Degrees of Influence Rule."

According to Christakis and Fowler (2009), everything we say or do can have a ripple effect among our sphere of influence, affecting our friends (one degree), our friends' friends (two degrees) and even the friends of our friends' friends (three degrees). According to their research, they have proven that the "three degrees rule of influence" applies to a broad range of behaviors and feelings as diverse as happiness, weight gain, and political views. In other words, your behavior can influence your friends' behaviors, your friends can influence their friends, and your friends' friends can influence their friends.

If we can influence people up to three degrees away from us, then one way to think about this is that each one of us has the ability to influence wide circles within our company, community, or network. For example, suppose you have 20 close contacts at work, which includes five colleagues, five peers, and ten other employees that you work with. Each of these people has the ability to influence a similar number of associates. As a result, you are indirectly connected to 400 other associates at two degrees of separation. But it doesn't stop there, it goes one step further (at three degrees) to the 20 associates they are connected to, yielding a total of $20 \times 20 \times 20$ people, or an amazing 8,000 individuals that are three degrees removed from you, which you can influence.

Thought of a little differently, a city with a population of two million people could theoretically be reached and influenced with the thoughts and behaviors of just 250 super engaged and influential people. Pretty amazing.

What Does this Mean to Food Safety?

The inferences from these studies are clear. They suggest that *food safety may be caught more than taught.*

Whether you realize it or not, having the proper attitude on food safety and demonstrating the right behaviors can influence thousands of individuals each day.

Think about the "Three Degrees of Influence" rule and how you might apply it to influence the organization where you work.

- For example, by working backwards from the total number of individuals you are trying to reach or influence, can you calculate the number of first degree people needed to create some sort of Food Safety Champion group? This group in turn can be used in a grassroots effort to reach or influence the next two degrees, for the total three degrees of influence.
- If you believe that food safety is not only taught but caught, consider identifying a group of "influencers" in your organization and intentionally getting them to model the proper food safety behaviors on a regular basis knowing that other people are watching and are likely to follow.
- What other ideas might you come up with?

Model, practice, and teach food safety on a daily basis within your sphere of influence. By working together with others, you can make a difference in an organization of any size, and make food safety the social norm and part of your organization's culture.

Chapter 19
Food Safety @ the Speed of Thought

Have you ever made a mistake, because you were in a hurry? For example, have you ever rushed to get an email sent and, after it had been sent and you re-read it, you caught grammatical errors that you had missed because you were in a rush. Of course you have.

While making a grammatical error in an email is not very significant, what if a doctor is in a hurry during a complicated surgery or an employee rushes while operating a dangerous piece of equipment? Do you think that could be risky or more prone to error?

Thinking Fast & Risk Taking Behavior

Previous research on this subject concludes that taking action or making decisions under time constraints leads to higher rates of error. This is somewhat intuitive. If you are rushed when performing an action or making a decision, it makes sense that you would be more likely to make a mistake, an error, or choose the wrong option.

However, two researchers, Chandler and Pronin (2012), wanted to look into this further. They wanted to know whether the 'momentary pace of one's own thoughts' affected risk-taking behaviors.

In their first experiment, they manipulated thought speed by having participants read trivia statements out loud at varying speeds. Afterwards, they assessed the participants' mood and their willingness to take risks. It turns out that those who were forced to read faster took more chances and increased their risk taking in a game with monetary payouts.

In a second experiment, Chandler and Pronin wanted to see if the risk taking behavior in the game translated to well-known behaviors like procrastinating, smoking marijuana, and engaging in unprotected sex. They induced fast, medium, and slow thought speeds by showing videos which had different angle shot lengths (0.75

© Springer Science+Business Media New York 2015
F. Yiannas, *Food Safety = Behavior*, Food Microbiology and Food Safety,
DOI 10.1007/978-1-4939-2489-9_19

s, 1.5 s, and 3 s). The length of the video clips were the same, the only difference was the speed of the shots. They then assessed risk taking behavior with a questionnaire which has been 'shown to predict risk-taking behavior.'

Intention to participate in risky behavior increased as the thought speed increased from slow to medium to fast in the video clip. In other words, those in the fast thinking group had the lowest perceptions of the negative consequences of risky behavior.

Of particular interest, these researchers determined through statistical analysis that it was 'thought speed' that resulted in mistakes and errors. Fast thought speed led to 'reduced consideration of the possible negative consequences,' which in turn led to increased risk-taking behavior.

They concluded two things from the study. First, thinking fast increases the positive mood of participants. They believe this could be due to some sort of physiological change in the brain, although they did not confirm this. Secondly, they concluded that thinking fast indirectly affects risk taking by decreasing the perception of negative consequences associated with the risky behavior.

The researchers draw implications for a wide range of situations: treatments designed to slow down the thought speed of manic patients could possibly decrease their risk taking behavior, slowing down your morning email reading could increase accurate decision making throughout the day, and, most provocatively, the video games and movies our youth enjoy could be increasing their risky behavior, *not* because of the content, but because of their *speed*.

What Does this Mean to Food Safety?

This research brings up dozens of questions for food safety research concerning potential applications to reduce risky food safety behaviors. Is it possible that the speed at which people "think" – not necessarily work – affects the decisions they make and thus their willingness to adopt risky behaviors when preparing food?

As an example of the potential application of this research, most food establishments have implemented a formal HACCP plan, which means that a competent authority has identified those points in the process – Critical Control Points (CCPs) – that if not controlled, could result in a foodborne outbreak. If the CCP is not highly automated and relies largely on human behavior (which many of them do), have you considered what else the employee has to do – and how fast they have to "think" at the time of conducting the CCP? This research suggests that we should not simply rely on Food Science to identify the CCP and how to reduce the hazard, but we should also utilize the Behavioral Sciences to see how likely the person executing the CCP might be to take shortcuts based on how quickly they are thinking. Having written and reviewed many HACCP plans, I find this to be quite an interesting and provocative thought.

Think about all of the processes in your work environment, especially at critical junctures that cause an employee to think fast (i.e., a rapidly changing menu screen at a cook station, multi-tasking that requires often changes in the direction of a person's thinking, etc.) and what they might mean to food safety. How can you intentionally design a barrier, which slows down the "thinking process" at these decisive junctures? Can you design some aspect of the environment, equipment, process, or tool, which forces the employee to slow down mentally at the critical control point?

Very importantly, please note that this research is not a criticism about working effectively and efficiently. In fact, in today's highly competitive world, being fast, effective, and efficient are one of the reasons companies remain successful in challenging times. However, in the area of food safety, while there may be a need to be fast, more importantly, we have to be safe and right.

Remember, this research shows that it is not necessarily the speed at which a person *works*, but the speed at which they *think* that might induce them to take risk-taking behaviors through a reduced perception of the consequences of such actions.

In closing, when it really counts, think slower, it could make the difference between safe and unsafe.

Chapter 20
Do Text Based Warning Labels Work?

I do not know about you, but at times it seems to me that society is starting to experience "warning label" fatigue. Think about the vast amount of products you can find in a store that have some sort of text-based warning label on them. Have you ever noticed them or have any caught your attention? More importantly, how often do any of these labels really influence your behavior?

While I realize that many of these labels may not be too important – and some are simply downright silly – there are others that really matter. For example, I think we all agree that warning labels on a product that is known to cause harm (i.e. cigarettes and alcohol) are a good idea. And while the intentions of such labels are right, at the end of the day, intentions do not really matter. Results do. Do these text based warning messages convey information in an effective manner and, more importantly, do they influence behavior? In other words, do they really work?

Changing Smoking Behaviors

Changing smoking behaviors is exactly what the government in the United Kingdom (UK) wanted to do. In the UK, it's been estimated that 100,000 deaths occur annually due to smoking-related deaths. In an attempt to discourage smoking, the Department of Health required that all cigarettes sold in the UK after October 2009 display graphic warning images on them.

Veer and Rank (2012) investigated the effectiveness of this policy by studying how the images impacted those trying to stop smoking, and if they kept others from taking up smoking. Although a few studies had previously suggested that graphic images are more effective than plain text warnings, the researchers wanted to probe the role the images play in a person's cognitive processing. The hypothesis being that challenges to a person's identity, in this case a smoker, would result in the person being more engaged with the thing challenging it.

© Springer Science+Business Media New York 2015
F. Yiannas, *Food Safety = Behavior*, Food Microbiology and Food Safety,
DOI 10.1007/978-1-4939-2489-9_20

Graphic Cigarette Warning Labels

The researchers chose to compare plain text-only warnings of the dangers of smoking with a graphic image-based warning label similar to those used by the UK with the accompanying text warning. After being shown a packet of cigarettes with either the plain text-only warning or the graphic image and text warning, participants were asked a series of questions concerning smoking behavior, their attention to the warning message, and their intentions to smoke (or start smoking). Lastly, they were given an assessment of smoking self-esteem (SSE) which relates the act of smoking to a person's level of self-esteem. Higher levels of SSE would suggest that an attack on smoking also is an attack on the smoker's worldview and, therefore, the smoker would be more likely to engage with the message.

An analysis of the study's results reveals that the difference between using graphic images and just text warnings on cognitive processing is significant. Cognitive processing relates to the process of thinking and remembering. On a 5 point Likert-scale, smokers experienced higher cognitive processing than nonsmokers (3.72 versus 3.00), but both were much higher than those shown just the text warnings (1.43 and 1.53 respectively). Participants who saw the visual warning label (graphic image) reported a much higher level of cognitive processing of the label than the text-only group, whose cognitive processing scores were extremely low.

For insights into the potential influence on behaviors, smokers indicated higher intentions to quit and nonsmokers not to start smoking as well when shown the graphic images (2.60 and 2.55 versus 2.07 and 2.28 respectively). Also of interest, those who indicated that they already had intentions to quit smoking were more influenced by the graphic labels than those who did not have prior intentions on quitting, suggesting that the images might remind them of the reality of the potential negative consequences of smoking.

What Does This Mean For Food Safety?

The implications of this research are clear and its potential applications to food safety are many. The use of graphic images could increase the cognitive processing (understanding and retention) of important food safety messages. While graphic images are rarely, if ever used in food safety, this research suggests that they might be a more effective way to reach various stakeholder groups (foodservice workers, consumers at home, etc.) than text based messages alone.

For example, when trying to ensure that food service workers and consumers fully cook their ground beef patties, could the use of graphic images help? In an employee training course, would a photo of a person's devastated kidney as a result of experiencing hemolytic uremic syndrome (HUS) due to an E. coli 0157:H7 infection obtained from an undercooked beef pattie enhance a person's understanding of the potentially severe consequences of not thoroughly cooking a hamburger? Would it further motivate their adherence to the cooking instructions on the label?

In the study, those who already were intending to quit smoking were more influenced by the graphic warnings than others. I wonder whether there is a corollary to food safety. For example, for food handlers and consumers who already know the right behaviors, but for some reason are not always in conformance with the desired behavior (using a thermometer, etc.), would graphic images of the potential consequences be the "nudge" they need to change their behavior?

Think about these findings and what they might mean to food safety. More research in this area, specifically applied to food safety, would be useful. And of course, we would want to do this in a thoughtful manner, so that we do not necessarily attack or discourage consumption of the food (ex. hamburger), but rather the unsafe behavior associated with its preparation (ex. undercooking).

In the meantime, remember this one important point. Images (potentially including graphic ones) are a more effective means of communication than all other forms of text-based methods. So, when communicating food safety, consider communicating with more than words.

Chapter 21
Enhancing Food Safety by Melody

Music, its everywhere. Have you ever stopped to think about this? For many of us, we wake up to the sound of music from our alarm clocks. We turn on the TV in the morning and there is background music on the news and in commercials. As we drive to work, we turn on the radio. Music permeates everything we do, and more importantly, it affects how we do it.

Music Affects Our Attitudes, Emotions, and Perceptions

I do not have to try to convince you that music can affect your attitude and emotions. I am sure you can relate to listening to a song that makes you happy, makes you sad, or even brings back warm and vivid memories.

More impressively, research by Logeswaran and Bhattacharya (2009) demonstrates that music can even affect our perceptions. In an experiment they conducted, 30 subjects were asked to listen to a series of happy or sad musical snippets. After listening to them, the research subjects were shown a photograph of a face. Some of the images contained a picture of a person with a happy face, and some contained a person with a sad or neutral facial expression. The research subjects were then asked to rate the perceived emotional content of the face on a scale ranging from 1 to 7 (1=extremely sad, 7=extremely happy).

The study found that the type of music the participant listened to prior to seeing the images significantly influenced the emotional ratings they gave to the faces they observed. In other words, music influenced their perceptions. In general, listening to happy music made happy faces appear to be even happier. And listening to sad music exaggerated the melancholy appearance of a frown.

While it probably seems obvious that music can evoke emotions, can it also influence behavior, especially safety-related behavior?

© Springer Science+Business Media New York 2015

F. Yiannas, *Food Safety = Behavior*, Food Microbiology and Food Safety, DOI 10.1007/978-1-4939-2489-9_21

Background Music and Safe Driving Behaviors

Brodsky and Slor (2013) wanted to know just that. They decided to study whether listening to one's preferred music style influenced driver safety versus listening to a generalized set of music. In other words, does your comfort level with the style of music being played affect your driving safety?

Eighty-five novice drivers (average age of 17.6 years old) were recruited, of whom only 8 % reported being involved in a collision previously. Asked about their musical preference while driving, almost all reported driving to music described as moderately-fast to very-fast paced and moderately-loud to loud (99 % and 94 % respectively). They were also asked to provide a CD of their preferred music while driving.

The researchers employed two well-experienced driving instructors to run driving evaluations. During six evaluations, the young drivers were evaluated according to driving safety actions and the number of times that the instructor had to intervene to prevent an immediate accident. For two evaluations, the driver's preferred music was played for 40 min (out of about 50 total minutes driving per session), for two evaluations a standard set of music was played (instrumental only; the clip the researchers provide on their website reminds me of light jazz), and for the other two evaluations there was no music played at all. In addition, the drivers were later evaluated for mood and impulsivity and sensation-seeking (something associated with driving).

While you might have predicted that participants would be more aware, or pay more attention to the non-familiar music being heard while driving, the reverse was true. Participants reported being more aware of the music while driving when it was their preferred music. In the assessment of impulsivity and sensation-seeking, the drivers could be segmented into two groups: those with high scores of impulsivity and sensation-seeking and those with low scores.

While all drivers reported having more positive moods when driving, their preferred music increased their positive mood versus driving with the alternative music set or without any music at all. Furthermore, this effect was more distinct in those participants with high impulsivity and sensation-seeking scores.

In evaluating the number of drivers that had at least one driving violation for each music type, the researchers determined that there appeared to be statistically significant differences: 90 % occurred with the alternative music, 95 % without music, and 98 % with their preferred music.

In evaluating the severity of the driving violations (failure to properly adjust speed, failure to stop, etc.) on a scaled rating system, preferred music resulted in the least attention paid to driving (6.66), alternative music resulted in the most attention (3.94), and no music was in between (5.15).

In summary, drivers liked listening to their preferred music and had a more positive mood while doing so, as opposed to no music or an alternative music type. However, drivers who listened to their preferred music experienced an increased number of safety violations. In multiple categories of assessment, providing an alternative music source actually decreased violations as compared to having no music at all.

What Does This Mean to Food Safety?

In many establishments that prepare food, ranging from food processing establishments to full-service restaurants to fast-food chains, it is not uncommon to allow employees to bring in their own radios and let them listen to their preferred music. However, these studies raise some interesting questions concerning the influence of music choice on food handlers, and its potential effects on food safety.

Below is a list of questions to consider and to potentially research further.

- Does the choice of background music influence an employee's adherence to desired food safety behaviors by distracting them or helping them focus attention? The research suggests music may help or hurt adherence.
- What is the overall effect of music on a group of food handlers with heterogeneous backgrounds, cultures, and preferences? Is there one-style of music that might be ideal to help keep a culturally diverse work staff focused on desired food safety behaviors?
- Considering that a food handler's duties can vary widely based on their position, could there be some positions that are more susceptible to musical distractions than others?

In closing, while some food establishments often put significant thought into what background music they play and how it influences the customer's shopping or dining experience, this research suggests we should also be as deliberate in choosing what type of music we allow our employees to listen to in the kitchen.

When it comes to food safety, details matter. And the research suggests that desired food safety behaviors might be enhanced by one's choice of melody.

Chapter 22
Can the Words We Use Influence Risk Perception?

The words we use matter. Why are they so important? It's because words have power. Words have started wars. They have helped nations make peace. They have influenced millions to take up great causes. They have made people believe in something bigger than themselves. They have sparked innovation. They have helped solved problems. Words can hurt. They can encourage. They can help educate.

If words are so powerful, then certainly they can be used to enhance food safety, right? Of course they can. They certainly play a critical role in ensuring our messages are clear and easily understood. In fact, have you ever noticed that gifted communicators tend to go farther in the workplace, are more likely to be listened to, and are more likely to be influential than others?

Despite the obvious benefits of effective communication, can the words we use actually influence a person's perception of risk and, in turn, their behavior?

Hard or Easy to Pronounce Fictitious Food Additives

The answer to this question lies in a study conducted by two behavioral science researchers (Song and Schwarz 2009). In their study, these researchers set up an experiment where they presented participants with a list of perceived ostensible food additives, containing either hard or easy to pronounce names. They then asked study participants to rank how risky they thought the food additives were to human health. How do you think the study participants rated the food additives based on their pronunciation?

Study participants perceived food additives with difficult to pronounce names, such as hnegripitrom, to be more harmful than food additives with easier to pronounce names, such as magnalroxate. Given that the study participants did not know that all of the ostensible food additives they were asked to rate were in fact all given names that were made up, these findings provide fascinating insight into the role

© Springer Science+Business Media New York 2015
F. Yiannas, *Food Safety = Behavior*, Food Microbiology and Food Safety,
DOI 10.1007/978-1-4939-2489-9_22

that fluency plays in the perception of risk. In other words, people believed that *if it was hard to pronounce, it must be riskier or more dangerous*. The bottom line is that by themselves, fluency and familiarity can influence a person's perception of risk.

Song and Scharz reached this same conclusion through a similar study of amusement rides. Participants who rode rides with hard to pronounce names perceived them to be more adventurous than rides that had more easily pronounceable names.

In summary, these studies suggest that the ease of pronunciation of names or terms influences one's perception of risk.

What Does This Mean to Food Safety?

The inferences from these studies suggest that a term's fluency (simplicity) or perceived similarity may influence ones perception of the risk of the stimuli, whether the stimuli is desirable or undesirable. This is noteworthy in the field of food safety for several reasons.

- **Risk perception influences behavior**. As indicated in the Health Belief Model of behavioral change by Janz et al. (2002), an individual's perception of risk is a good predictor of their likelihood to engage in health promoting behaviors. By simply naming something with an easy or hard to pronounce name, its conceivable that we can influence a person's risk perception and, in turn, their behavior.
- **Hard to pronounce work processes and technologies might be perceived to be risky**. There is no question about it, to dramatically advance food safety and to feed a growing global population, we need new and innovative food technologies. However, these research findings suggest that what researchers name these technologies is more important than we think. Even if a technology is safe and holds great promise to promote a safer global food supply in the future, if the technology is given a name that is hard to pronounce or unfamiliar, it is likely to be perceived as risky and possibly rejected. As a classic example, surveys have shown that consumers respond to the term "genetically modified foods" with concern and often avoid foods with this label. On the other hand, consumers are much more likely to accept and try a food described as being produced using "biotechnology" – although this is simply a different way to describe the exact same food production technique used in genetically modified foods.

In closing, think about these findings and how you might use them to enhance food safety. Remember, when deciding what to call a new work process, procedure, or technology, you better think twice: its name is much more important than you think. And it could make the difference between adoption and rejection.

Chapter 23
Don't Be a Food Safety Bystander

When observing an imminent or potentially hazardous situation (ranging from a medical emergency to a potential fire), how do you think the average person will respond? Do you think they are likely to help or, in contrast, do you think they are likely to go about their normal course of business as though the threat was unnoticed?

The answer to this question may surprise you, as it seems counter-intuitive.

In the mid 1960s, a young woman named Kitty Genovese was returning to her apartment in New York City when she was viciously attacked. After detectives investigated the attack, the *New York Times* ran a front page story (which is now well known in social science circles) on how a large number of respectable citizens witnessed or heard the attack, yet failed to help or call the police.

Two social psychologists working in New York at the time, Bibb Latane and John Darley, were deeply disturbed by this phenomena and set out to conduct a series of experiments to determine if there was a rationale that could explain it. The two researchers theorized that the number of observers may have played a pivotal role in why people behaved the way they did, so they set out to conduct a series of experiments to test their hypothesis.

Willingness to Help in a Medical Emergency

In one study, Latané and Darley (1968) had a student fake an epileptic seizure on a street in New York City and observed whether passers-by would stop to help. Since they were interested in exploring if the number of observers made a difference, they staged the fake seizure repeatedly in front of different sizes of crowds. The results were conclusive. As the number of witnesses increased, the chances that any single observer would help decreased. The student faking the seizure received assistance 85 % of the time when there was only one other person present. However, this

© Springer Science+Business Media New York 2015
F. Yiannas, *Food Safety = Behavior*, Food Microbiology and Food Safety,
DOI 10.1007/978-1-4939-2489-9_23

percentage dropped amazingly to 35 % of the time when five observers were present. The greater the number of people that observed the seizure, the less likely it was that any one person would help.

Where There Is Smoke, There Is Fire

In another study, Latané and Darley (1969) created another fake emergency scenario. In this experiment, they studied the response of people sitting in a waiting room to simulated smoke seeping under the door, suggesting that a fire had broken out in the building. Once again, the larger the group, the less likely that any single person in the waiting room would sound the alarm. In fact, when a single person was sitting in the waiting room, 75 % reported the smoke. Disturbingly, when there were three people in the waiting room, only 38 % reported the smoke.

This same pattern – the larger the group observing a serious situation, the less likely that any single person will do anything about it – has been proven in numerous behavioral science studies. Social psychologists now refer to this phenomenon as the "Bystander Effect." Behavioral scientists believe this phenomenon occurs because, among other reasons, individual observers all assume that someone else is going to intervene and do something about it, so each individual feels less responsible and refrains from doing anything.

What Does This Mean to Food Safety?

The implications from this research are clear. When it comes to food safety in today's interdependent food system or in an organization of any significant size, we cannot allow people to fall into the trap of the "Bystander Effect" mindset and assume that someone else will take care of food safety.

Of interest, the "Bystander Effect" can hinder all segments of the food system as well as various stakeholder groups. While I am sure you can think of more, below are just two examples of how a "Bystander Mindset" could hinder food safety.

- If you are a food producer that manufacturers a food product that has to be cooked, a "Bystander Mindset" could result in an over-reliance on assuming the final cook will inactivate any pathogens that might be present, rather than striving for continuous improvement and implementing new pathogen reduction interventions in the product being produced.
- In a large organization with dozens of individuals working in the same kitchen, a "Bystander Mindset" could result in some employees tolerating an unsanitary or unsafe condition, assuming someone else will fix it.

Remember that food safety is a shared responsibility, but its also a personal responsibility. Make sure that employees within your organization know specifically what it is that they have to do to produce safe food, and never assume others will take care of an unsafe condition.

Think about the "Bystander Effect" and what it might mean to you and your organization. And more importantly, think about what you can to do prevent it. Instead of the "Bystander Effect", help others adopt this mindset: Food Safety Begins with Me!

Chapter 24
To Checklist or Not to Checklist?

In this chapter, I wanted to share a few thoughts on a common crutch I often find many food safety professionals using. It's an over-reliance on checklists as the ultimate solution to a lack of compliance with desired behaviors, which is based on a misunderstanding of what checklists should and should not be used for.

To be an effective food safety professional, you must avoid developing an overly simplistic checklist mentality in hopes of driving behavior change. You see, I believe that by reducing food safety to a checklist, you could unintentionally create a mindset (and checklist culture) where employees are not really focused on what they need to do to produce safe food (the right behaviors), but rather make sure all the boxes are ticked off to show that they did food safety, when in many cases they did not.

Checklists Improve Healthcare Outcomes

Now, please do not get me wrong. I am not against checklists. There are times when checklists are needed and useful. In fact, Atul Gawande (2009), physician and author, does a wonderful job of reviewing how well-designed checklists can ensure desired behaviors and improve outcomes in medicine, ranging from dispensing the right medications to reducing infection rates in the surgical room.

For example, in a study on the usefulness of checklists conducted at John Hopkins University and summarized in Atul Gawande's book, *The Checklist Manifesto*, researchers calculated that infection rates associated with one particular procedure dropped from 11 % to 0 %. It was estimated that because of the use of one simple checklist – and the behaviors it induced – the hospital staff prevented 43 infections, 8 deaths, and saved approximately 2 million dollars in a little over 1 year.

There is no question about it. Properly designed checklist and their appropriate use can make a big difference. They can even save lives. However, before you

© Springer Science+Business Media New York 2015
F. Yiannas, *Food Safety = Behavior*, Food Microbiology and Food Safety,
DOI 10.1007/978-1-4939-2489-9_24

jump to the conclusion that a checklist is the right solution to achieve a particular outcome, a thorough needs assessment test should be performed. In other words, if a desired performance outcome is not being achieved, its critical to conduct a thoughtful analysis on why the desired outcome is not being met. Is it a lack of clear performance expectations? Do employees need to be better trained or educated? Is the work designed in an overly complex manner? Do employees have the right tools to enhance the likelihood of compliance? If these critical concepts are not properly addressed, no checklist can guarantee success. As an exaggerated example, imagine a scenario where a plane's cockpit is poorly designed and has poorly trained pilots. In this scenario, the checklist will not be able to fly the plane.

Lessons Learned from the Cockpit

Nowhere are checklists more frequently used for safety purposes than in the airline industry. And while checklists have been used by the airline industry for a long time, a search of the literature revealed that they really had not been studied well from a human behavioral standpoint. Accordingly, two researchers wanted to know just that, as the improper use or non-use of checklists by airline crew was often cited as a contributing factor in airline crashes.

Degani and Wiener (1993) wanted to look into when checklists were being used, how they were being used, and how they might be designed for greater effectiveness. In one section of their study involving field observations, the researchers actually sat in the cockpit observer's seat and watched checklist usage in one major U.S. airline. For their study, the researchers observed 42 flight crews on 72 short to mid range fights for 140 total hours of flight time. To not bias the results, the cockpit crews were never told why the observers were present, nor did the researchers take any notes or make any comments during the flights.

A summary of their observations is revealing and sheds valuable insight into how checklists are used and how they might be better designed. Two repeated observations in particular are worthy of mention. First, in several instances, pilots never even pulled the checklists out of their protective sleeves. Instead, they performed the checks from memory. Clearly, this increases the chance that a step might be overlooked. Second, several pilots were observed doing what the researchers called "short-cutting." When checklists were long, rather than doing one check at a time and in the desired order, several pilots would actually perform several checks together for expediency, in other words "chunk them" and note them afterwards collectively as having been completed. Clearly, this is in stark contrast to the intended purpose of the checklist and relies on the pilot's short and long-term memory to ensure that the critical checks were truly conducted.

What Does This Mean to Food Safety?

The findings from this research are interesting and certainly have direct implications for food safety. Food safety professionals and food safety plans commonly use checklists as a means to ensure adherence to certain procedures, behaviors, and conditions. However, like the airline industry, a review of the literature reveals that their use in food safety has not been well studied.

The research above reminds us that not all checklists are created equal. There are both good and bad checklists. According to Atul Gawande, *"Bad checklists are vague and imprecise."* In contrast, Atul states, *"Good checklists are precise. They do not try to spell out everything. Instead, they provide reminders of only the most critical and important steps."*

With this thought in mind and based on research from other industries, let me briefly share a few tips on what a checklist *should* and *should not* be used for.

A Checklist **should** be used:

- As an instructional "read – do" approach for highly complex tasks that are not frequently performed to ensure the critical steps are properly followed and none are accidently missed or overlooked.
- As a "do – confirm" approach for critical tasks to verify and document that key steps have been taken and that they conform to critical performance standards. In fact, this is how checklists are most commonly used in the field of food safety under the Hazardous Analysis of Critical Control Point (HACCP) approach – making sure those Critical Control Points, also known as CCPs (i.e. cooking, hot holding, cold holding) are checked at certain frequencies throughout the day to ensure that they are under control, and documenting that those critical checks have taken place.

A Checklist **should not** be used:

- To replace clear performance expectations, training and education of employees, effective design of work-processes, or proper equipment and work tools.
- For very simple tasks with low criticality or low complexity.

In closing, remember that creating a checklist is easy. The harder part is discerning if a checklist is really needed, what to check (frequency, critical limits, etc.), how to design it so that its used correctly and, very importantly, how to use the information it provides to improve food safety.

Chapter 25
The Most Powerful Word in Food Safety

If someone were to ask you, what is the most powerful word in the English language that you can use to enhance food safety, what would your answer be?

Please pause, take a minute to think about it, and write down or remember the one word you would choose.

What was your answer? Did you write down the acronym "HACCP" or words "law" or "regulation?" How about the words "priority" or "responsibility?" Some with a more punitive mindset may have said "punishment" or "fines." Although they are all common answers, approaches, and "words," in my opinion, they all miss the mark.

Think about it. As a food safety professional, the production of safe food is largely about getting others to say "yes" to your requests. In fact, food safety professionals are trying to get others to say "yes" in an attempt to manage food safety every day. For example, you may ask others to consistently adhere to a desired practice or behavior, such as taking required food temperatures, washing their hands, or adhering to proper sanitation procedures. At other times, you might be trying to get buyers to say "yes" and only do business with suppliers that meet certain food safety requirements or get senior management to invest in new equipment or process changes.

Bottom line, food safety professionals are always in the business of trying to get others to say YES. With this thought in mind, is there a single word – more important than any other – that can enhance your ability to get others to say "yes?"

Moving to the Head of the Line

The answer to this question lies in a simple behavioral study conducted by researchers at Harvard University a few years ago. In the study, researchers went to the college library at a time of day when they knew there was always a long line of

© Springer Science+Business Media New York 2015   89
F. Yiannas, *Food Safety = Behavior*, Food Microbiology and Food Safety,
DOI 10.1007/978-1-4939-2489-9_25

individuals waiting to use the copy machine. They then tested three different scenarios. In the first scenario, one of the experimenters would walk to the front of the long line of students waiting to make copies and ask, *can I cut to the front of the line*? If you were in this line, what would you do? Would you let another student ahead of you after you had been patiently waiting your turn? Amazingly, 60 % of the test subjects (students in the line) that were asked the question let a random stranger cut to the front of the line.

In the second scenario, the researcher would walk to the front of the line at the copy machine, but this time they asked the question differently. Rather than simply asking, can I cut to the front of the line, they also provided a reason. Specifically, they asked, *can I cut to the front of the line because I'm in a hurry and late for class*? Under this scenario, where a reason was given, what do you think happened? Compliance with this request increased, with 94 % of the test subjects letting a random stranger cut to the front of the line. In other words, with little to no effort, compliance increased a whopping 34 % by simply asking the question a little differently. Asking someone to do something is not good enough. The way you ask matters tremendously. People generally want to know the reason or the "why" behind the request you have made of them. You can get greater compliance if you provide the reason – and the word "because" provides the perfect cue that a rationale is forthcoming.

The study gets even more interesting. In a third scenario, the researcher would go to the front of the line, ask the question if they could cut in front, but they provided a rationale that was much weaker. In this scenario, they asked, *can I cut to the front of the line because I have to make copies*? Clearly, this is not a very convincing reason. Everyone standing in the line presumably has to make copies. Faced with this situation, how would you respond? Amazingly, a whopping 93 % of the test subjects in this scenario still let a random stranger cut to the front of the line, suggesting that the mere use of a reason, even if it's a weak one, might enhance the likelihood of compliance.

What Does This Mean to Food Safety?

The results of this study suggest that when food safety professionals ask employees to adopt a new practice or desired behavior, simply asking is not enough. Always explain the "why" when making your request. In my experience, food safety professionals are very good about the "what" and the "how," but this simple research study reminds us that the "why" matters. And it matters a lot. People are much more likely to comply, understand, and buy-in, if you provide a rationale as to why you are making the request. Always take the time to provide a convincing rationale or reason on why you are asking people to do things.

Therefore, the most powerful word in the English language to enhance food safety could very well be the word *because*, as it requires us to explain the "why" or the reason behind our request. Keep this word in your mental back pocket as a reminder to always explain the "why" behind your requests.

In closing, think about the various requests you make of employees to adhere to food safety, whether it's through training, SOPs, or other means. Are you doing enough to explain the "why?" Explaining the "why" behind your request is likely to significantly increase the chances of getting others to say YES to food safety.

Chapter 26
Food Safety in Mind through Building Design

How much influence does a building's architect and designer have on your behavior? Could they influence you to do something out of your normal routine while you are in the building? It turns out that we all might be more susceptible to a building's architectural influence than we might realize.

Influencing Behavior by Design

Retailers in particular know that a store's design can influence shopper behavior and movement. For example, studies have shown that when a store lay-out follows a racetrack form, a large percentage of shoppers can be influenced to follow the designed path with little thought due to the store's layout (Levy and Weitz 1998).

Food safety professionals also know the importance of building design and its influence on behaviors. For example, it's common for food safety professionals to intentionally design a physical separation between areas that contain raw meat and those in which ready-to-eat foods are handled in order to minimize the potential for cross-contamination.

Collective Effects of Building Intent

However, a few researchers, Wu et al. (2013), wanted to look at building design in a broader sense. They wanted to know whether "contextual factors" about building design at an "aggregate level" would affect pro-environmental or sustainable behavior.

© Springer Science+Business Media New York 2015
F. Yiannas, *Food Safety = Behavior*, Food Microbiology and Food Safety,
DOI 10.1007/978-1-4939-2489-9_26

In other words, they wanted to know whether the fact that the entire building, not just individual aspects, was designed for sustainability would influence pro-sustainability behaviors.

To do this, they decided to study whether patrons correctly disposed of their lunch trash into one of three bins in a café area: garbage, compostable, and recycling. They chose to use the café in the Centre for Interactive Research on Sustainability (CIRS) at the University of British Columbia, because the building was explicitly designed for sustainability – what they describe as "designed with intent." For a control, they chose the student union's (SUB) food court. Both buildings were used because they already had all three disposal bins in place.

In both buildings, two people discretely observed patrons at the discarding bins. The goal was to note whether items were being discarded properly. For example, if a bottle and napkin were both placed in the recycling bin, the bottle would be marked as correct but the napkin, which should have been composted, as incorrect. After the observation period, the two people compared notes to ensure that all of the actions were observed correctly.

It turns out that 86 % of disposal events in CIRS were properly made as opposed to only 58 % in SUB. That's an almost 30 % difference in behavior!

The researchers recognized that it could have been possible that the people eating in CIRS were there because they worked there and, thus, they might already be inclined to act sustainably. This would be a sampling bias and cause skewed results. Therefore, they surveyed patrons at both CIRS and SUB, finding that only one person actually worked in CIRS and that many at CIRS frequently ate at SUB and vice versa. In addition, while patrons rated sustainability as a reason to eat at CIRS, they rated it below convenience. In this way, they eliminated the question of whether there was a sampling bias.

Lastly, they wanted to determine "why" the difference in behavior existed, despite the fact that each café was set up identically with three disposal bins each: garbage, compostable, and recycling. The researchers speculated that it was due to an effect known as "embodied cognition." In short, embodied cognition states that the context in which we find ourselves affects the way we perceive and behave. They asked patrons in both buildings "how environmentally conscious they thought they were in their current building." On a scale from 1 to 5, patrons in CIRS had an average of 3.58 versus patrons in SUB that had an average of 2.92.

It seems that the pro-sustainability behavior correlated with building awareness.

What Does This Mean to Food Safety?

The findings from this research could have direct implications for food safety, worker safety, and numerous other areas. As such, we should pause to consider them.

First, in the study referenced above, simply being in the CIRS building raised an individual's conscious awareness about sustainability and, in turn, their pro-sustainability related behaviors. This is amazing and powerful.

Secondly, the building drew a patron's attention to the sustainable features in it. This is distinctly different from the situation when the building's design intentionally and physically guides a patron to a particular or desired behavior. Again, since both buildings in the study had the same waste disposal bins, the behavior changes were not due to the physical constraints of the building. Instead, it was the totality of the building's environment. In other words, the effect was not due to a single element, but due to the building having been "designed with intent."

The research suggests that when we think about designing a retail food establishment or a food manufacturing facility, we might just need a paradigm shift. Instead of simply designing food safety components into the building, we should instead design the building with food safety intent. These are two different motivations. Moreover, the study also indicates that we should think about ways to raise awareness and draw our employee's attention to the food safety design features of the building, rather than keeping silent about them.

I encourage you to think about these findings and what they might mean to food safety. For example:

- If we have two buildings designed similarly, would explicitly telling employees about the food safety design elements increase the positive behavior change?
- Which food safety design features in your establishment are most attention grabbing? Are there enough of them and do the employees in your building know about them? If not, maybe they should be a topic for new employees during orientation.
- Conversely, are there design features that seem in conflict with food safety and therefore could decrease awareness and suppress desired behaviors?

In closing, while building architects and designers often go to great lengths to comply with a health department's plan review requirements, this research suggests that maybe we should do more. Not only is it critical that we specifically and intentionally design buildings with food safety in mind, we also should raise awareness of all the collective food safety design features of the building and promote their awareness. In other words, we might be able to keep food safety in mind by raising awareness of building design.

Chapter 27
Does How You Make a Food Safety Request Matter?

As a food safety and compliance professional, your success often depends on getting others to say yes to your requests. For example, you may be asking associates to follow specific procedures or adhere to a set of desired, safe behaviors. Knowing that your success depends on others saying "yes," how much time do you spend thinking about the manner in which you will ask others to comply with your requests?

Is your approach based on proven behavioral science techniques or is it merely based on your opinion, which has been established through trial and error?

Insight into how to ask others to comply with your requests can be gleaned from a study conducted by Flynn and Bohns (2010). In a field study they conducted at New York's Penn Station, people were approached by an experimenter and asked to fill out a two-page questionnaire.

In the first study group, targets were asked, "will you fill out a questionnaire?" In the second study group, targets were first asked, "can you do me a favor?" – before hearing the same request – "will you fill out a questionnaire?"

Interestingly, 57 % of the targets in the first group complied with filling out the questionnaire. In the second group, when asked first, "will you do me a favor?" – compliance increased to a whopping 84 %. Even more dramatically, when the experimenter paused and allowed the target subject's in the second group to say "yes," compliance in completing the form increased to nearly 100 %.

This study demonstrates the powerful influence of commitment inducing requests. In other words, this study is consistent with behavioral scientist Robert Cialdini's principle of commitment (1993). Getting others to say yes to an initial smaller request increases the chances of them saying yes to a later, larger requests.

© Springer Science+Business Media New York 2015
F. Yiannas, *Food Safety = Behavior*, Food Microbiology and Food Safety,
DOI 10.1007/978-1-4939-2489-9_27

What Does This Mean to Food Safety?

The inference from this study is clear. It indicates that merely making a request for others to comply with food safety in the "right way" can make a dramatic difference in the degree to which others will say yes.

Think about how an inspector might use this finding to strengthen compliance in the facility they are inspecting. For example, it's not uncommon for inspectors and auditors to give instructions on what needs to be fixed while conducting an audit. However, this research suggests the way they make those requests matter. By being mindful of the power of commitment inducing scripts, with something as simple as, will you do me a favor?; they'll be much more likely to persuade others to action.

Although society teaches us that the most important thing to say is "please" prior to making such requests, objective research data tells us something different. Although good manners are always a good idea and appreciated, getting others to make a small commitment first might hold the key to success. Something as simple as an initial question, such as "would you please do me a favor?" and pausing to get an affirmative response, could make the difference between success and failure.

Chapter 28
Is the Sum of Food Safety Efforts Greater Than In Parts?

In this chapter, I would like to share thoughts on one of the topics most frequently discussed in business and sports – teamwork. Strictly defined, teamwork is *the coordinated effort on the part of a group of persons acting together as a team or in the interests of a common cause.* Clearly, committed individuals working together can achieve more than by just working alone. That is why teamwork is so important. This point was stated well by Michael Jordan, one of the NBA's greatest players of all time, who said, *"Talent wins games, but teamwork wins championships."*

However, does working on a team guarantee greater productivity or better results?

To answer this question, I would like to share the results of a research study conducted by Max Ringelmann (1913). Dr. Ringelmann is well known in social science circles for conducting a series of experiments in which he measured individual and group performance on a series of rope-pulling tasks. One would expect that when placed in a group, a team's collective rope-pulling efforts would be at least equal to, if not greater than, the sum of the individual abilities of each person in that group. For example, three people pulling together on the rope should exert three times as much force as a single person; eight people should exert eight-times as much force, and so on.

However, much to his surprise, Dr. Ringelmann's study did not confirm this expectation at all. His research instead demonstrated that groups of three people pulling together exerted a force equivalent to two-and-a-half times the average individual's performance. Oddly, the larger the group, the less they achieved. Groups of eight people collectively pulling together on the rope exerted a force less than four times the average individual rate. The conclusions from this research have been replicated by behavioral scientists in similar experiments, which confirm that increases in group size are inversely related to individual effort or performance.

You might be asking yourself, how can this be? Why would a group's effort result in less than the sum of the individual efforts combined?

© Springer Science+Business Media New York 2015
F. Yiannas, *Food Safety = Behavior*, Food Microbiology and Food Safety,
DOI 10.1007/978-1-4939-2489-9_28

Psychologists theorize that some individuals may expend less effort when working together with others as a team as compared to when they work alone. For example, if responsibility is dispersed amongst a group, an individual, realizing that his contribution cannot be accurately measured, may be tempted to ride on the coat-tails of everyone else's efforts. Behavioral psychologists have termed this *social loafing*.

What Does This Mean to Food Safety?

If you think about it, although there is no question that the emergence of today's modern food system has provided consumers with a more diverse food supply and convenient source of prepared, economical, and ready-to-eat meals, these trends have resulted in both benefits and additional risks. Today's food system requires more "interdependence" by multiple stakeholders and points in the food continuum (farmers, transporters, importers, retailers, consumers, etc.) than ever before. In fact, never before in history has the concept of shared responsibility for food safety been more important than it is today.

Even within a single company, food safety is a shared responsibility (which requires teamwork) dependent on many individuals doing their part – ranging from buyers, warehouse personnel, truck drivers, operational managers, maintenance personnel, food safety professionals, and front-line employees. Each person within a company has a personal responsibility to ensure that the work they do enables the organization to deliver safe food. Consequently, the sum of food safety efforts within an organization is critically dependent on and, ideally, greater than its parts. A food safety management system will only be as strong as its weakest link.

However, this research, based on the concept of social loafing, suggests that the greater the number of individuals involved in producing food, whether it be in a single manufacturing plant or along the entire food continuum, the more likely it is that some individuals will not do their part – believing that their contribution to the process (or lack thereof) may not be seen or noticed.

Think about the concept of social loafing as it relates to stakeholders in the food system or employees in your organization, and what it might mean to food safety. Realize that social loafing is a product of human nature and create systems to prevent it.

For example, by understanding the concept of social loafing, can we create systems that decrease the anonymity of any individual's efforts and ensure that the sum of collective efforts is at least equal to its parts? Clearly defined food safety objectives with measurable outcomes at each point (and for each segment) in the food continuum is a great way to deter social loafing and make sure everyone does their part. Anything that allows us to witness or measure individual contributions is a good place to start in our efforts to deter social loafing.

In closing, do your part to help others believe that food safety is not only a shared responsibility, but a personal responsibility as well. Additionally, get all employees in the organization to adopt a mindset that Food Safety, It Begins with Me!

Chapter 29
Making Food Safety Fun

Can food safety be fun? I know, some food safety purist will say that food safety is not about having fun. Its about personal responsibility. And yes, you are absolutely right!

But remember, at the end of the day, what a group of employees or individuals know about food safety principles or what they think or believe about food safety is of less importance than what they do – their behavior is critically important.

So how can we help shape or reinforce desired food safety behaviors? One of the most important ways to do so is through the proper use of consequences. That is right – consequences. And "fun" might just be a very effective consequence in influencing certain desired behaviors. It certainly will not work in all circumstances, but it could be one of the many tools we use to try to influence desired behaviors.

The Fun Theory

The carmaker Volkswagen has been promoting an idea called the Fun Theory. Its based on the idea that an idea as simple as having fun can be used to change people's behavior for the better. Volkswagen has been using this idea to promote car safety. However, the theory can be applied to improve behaviors that are better for you, the environment, or – in our case – food safety.

The World's Deepest Garbage Bin

To promote the Fun Theory, Volkswagen sponsored a series of contests where people could submit their ideas on how to make desired, socially responsible behaviors fun. One of the award winners came up with an idea regarding litter.

© Springer Science+Business Media New York 2015 101
F. Yiannas, *Food Safety = Behavior*, Food Microbiology and Food Safety,
DOI 10.1007/978-1-4939-2489-9_29

If you think about it, something as simple as throwing trash (or as the British say, rubbish) into a bin instead of on the ground can be challenging. Despite the focus on taking care of the environment, how many people still fail to do so? All you have to do is visit any park, outdoor market, stadium, etc., and you will see that littering is still a big social problem (especially in certain regions of the country and world).

With this theory in mind, one Volkswagen contestant wanted to know if they could get people to throw their garbage in trash bins by making it fun.

To do so, they decided to design the world's deepest garbage bin. They took a real trash bin already being used in a park and designed it to create an audible noise that sounded like something falling a very, very long distance whenever people threw trash into the bin. To hear and see how it worked, watch the YouTube video titled "the World's Deepest Bin" (The Fun Theory 2001).

In a simple experiment conducted in a well-established city park, the world's deepest garbage bin collected 72 kg of garbage. To put that into perspective: that amount was 41 kg more trash than was collected in a non-audible bin just a short distance away. In other words, by making the behavior of throwing away trash fun, the researchers were able to almost double the amount of trash collected in one bin in just one day!

Positive Consequences Eat Negative Ones for Lunch

While the example above emphasizes fun, the reality is that this has more to do with "positive consequences" than it does fun. As stated by B.F. Skinner, *"the consequence of an act affects the probability of it occurring again."*

Every single day, people do things because of potential consequences. Yes, the consequences of an act affect the probability of it occurring again. For example, if we do something that produces a consequence that we like or that benefits us (like getting recognized or rewarded for a certain behavior), we are more likely to do it again. If we do something that produces a consequence that we do not like or that does not benefit us (like burning our hand on a hot stove), we are less likely to do it again.

When trying to influence human behavior, its important to have the right balance between positive consequences and negative consequences. However, studies have repeatedly shown that emphasis on positive consequences over negative consequences generally leads to enhanced performance and results. For example, Madesen and Madsen (1974) found that teachers who used positive reinforcement over negative at a ratio of at least 4 to 1 were able to achieve higher performance and discipline in their classrooms. There are numerous other studies that have demonstrated this same principle. For enhanced performance and results, the frequency of positive consequences should significantly outweigh the use of negative consequences. That is why the Fun Theory works so well.

What Does This Mean to Food Safety?

The implications from this research are extremely relevant to food safety. If consequences can help increase desired or decrease undesired behaviors, then certainly they can be used to enhance food safety performance, right? Of course they can.

Thought of a little differently, if an organization is not seeing improvements in food safety, then one contributing factor may be that they are not effectively using consequences to manage performance. Organizations that are able to meet specific and objective food safety goals year after year and improve food safety performance most likely have figured out a way to develop effective consequences. And those that are maximizing the use of positive consequences are likely to be best in class.

Think about the use of positive consequences, the Fun Theory, and how they might be used to reinforce select, desired behaviors. For example:

*   Would making hand washing fun, especially in school or other settings where kids have to wash their hands, help children adopt good hand washing practices? Moreover, could it leave a lasting, positive imprint on the child, and thereby affect hand-washing behavior for their entire life?
*   In the workplace, are there certain desired behaviors you could influence for the better by making them fun? As an example, one thing food processing plants often want is for employees in boots to walkthrough a footbath and ensure that their boots make contact with a sanitizing solution for a brief period of time. What if the footbath activates a fun song only when the boot has been in contact with the bath for the desired period of time? Would this ensure footbath practices were properly followed? One could change the tune of the song periodically to keep up the sense of novelty.

I am sure that you can come up with a list of your own ideas and I hope you do. More importantly, try putting one into practice.

And remember, these wise words given by Dr. Michael LeBoeuf in his book, *The Greatest Management Principle in the World* (1985): "Managers don't get what they hope for, train for, beg for, or even demand. Managers get what they recognize and reward through positive consequences."

Chapter 30
Role Modeling Food Safety

Have you ever stopped to think about the power of role models in our society, community, place of work, or even in your own life? Think about it. Are there role models that have influenced you in a profound way? I suspect there are, as role models have a powerful influence on the behaviors of others, whether for good or bad.

A role model is defined as a person who serves in a particular behavioral or social role for another person to emulate. Another good definition is that a role model is a person regarded by others as a good example to follow.

And guess what, role models are everywhere. Role models can range from celebrities and the influences they have on the clothing selections others make, to the athlete that influences others on her team and kids all across the nation. There are role models in the classroom, political circles, and, yes, even at work.

If role models are so powerful at influencing others, can they be used to strengthen food safety in an organization? In other words, can an organization increase its compliance by intentionally and very specifically modeling desired food safety related behaviors or tasks? Of course it can! Let me share just one example of the powerful effect role modeling can have on compliance behaviors.

Influencing Others to Wash Their Hands

In public health settings as well as in food establishments, one of the most basic, yet important behaviors workers have to comply with is hand washing. Yet as simple as it sounds, it can be a big struggle to get employees to comply, even when they are highly trained medical professionals.

In such settings, a factor that is perceived as a barrier to better hand hygiene compliance is a lack of access to conveniently located hand sinks. In fact, over the years, health departments have required more and more hand sinks to be installed in

© Springer Science+Business Media New York 2015   105
F. Yiannas, *Food Safety = Behavior*, Food Microbiology and Food Safety,
DOI 10.1007/978-1-4939-2489-9_30

hospital settings and in retail food establishments. Another factor often perceived as a barrier to better hand hygiene compliance is a lack of time, with some suggesting that when workers are too busy, they will not stop to wash their hands. One well known company even went as far as having an audible alarm go off every 30 min to remind employees to stop and wash their hands, as though this might be the key to better hand washing compliance.

While these perceptions have been around for years and are still held by many public health professionals, there is really little evidence to indicate that they play an important role in hand washing.

More Hand Wash Sinks or More Role Models

Lankford et al. (2003) wanted to investigate what really motivates a person to wash their hands. Is there a correlation between having a hand sink that is conveniently located, functional, and properly designed with good hand washing compliance? Or are other factors – non-physical in nature – more important?

To investigate this, the researchers selected two hospitals (one old, one new) in which to observe hand washing behaviors among hospital staff. In the old hospital, the hand sink to bed ratio ranged from 8 hand sinks for every 33 rooms to 4 hand sinks for every 23 rooms, depending on which department in the hospital you were in. In stark contrast, the new hospital had a hand sink to bed ratio of 1 to 1. In other words, there was a hand sink in every single patient's room.

In the study, the researchers defined a hand hygiene event as a worker washing their hands with soap and water for any length of time. Moreover, no other types of hand hygiene alternatives (such as hand sanitizers) were available for the study. Importantly, while the workers knew there was a new person working with them (the researcher), they did not know that they were there to make observations on hand washing practices, so that they would not base their behavior on the researcher's presence.

Between both hospitals, the researchers made a total of 45 h of hand washing observations. Over that course of time, a total of 305 hand washing opportunities were made in the old hospital, and a total of 424 were made in the new hospital. Observations were made on select hospital workers, with the majority including nurses and physicians.

The Findings

While one might expect that compliance with hand washing should be dramatically better in the new hospital (after all, they had a hand sink in every room!) this was not the case. Surprisingly, hand washing compliance prior to or upon room entry was significantly greater in the old hospital (12 %) compared to at the new hospital

(6 %). In fact, the overall ratio of hand washing compliance to defined opportunities was significantly better at the old hospital compared to the new (53 % vs. 23 %)

Of even greater interest, a multivariate analysis of a variety of issues identified that the most important factor in whether a person washed their hands was not the presence of a conveniently located hand sink. Instead, it was discovered that health care workers in a room where a peer or higher-ranking worker did not wash their hands were significantly less likely to wash their hands as well. The researchers concluded that the effect of a role model is highly significant and most potent in negatively influencing hand washing behavior.

In summary, while some regulatory officials and professionals might believe that access to conveniently located and well-designed hand sinks is the most important factor in hand washing compliance, this research clearly demonstrates that this assumption, although well intentioned, is flawed.

What Does This Mean to Food Safety?

The inferences from this research go far beyond hand washing and can relate to a wide variety of food safety and compliance-related issues (taking food temperatures, wearing personal protective equipment, etc.). While facility design, equipment selection, and work tools are important factors to consider when attempting to strengthen compliance, they are not always sufficient to explain why workers accept or reject certain behaviors. Behavior is more complex than that. Often times, in order to shape and achieve the desired behavior, we need to consider more than just the physical elements. We need to model the desired behavior ourselves.

Think about the research findings and what they might mean to a particular practice or behavior in the workplace that you want to improve. Ask yourself:

- Is the desired behavior being modeled enough by other employees in similar positions? If its not, the research suggests it will be hard for others to adopt the behavior.
- Conversely, can you create a strategy around the specific, desired behavior and convince champions in the organization, especially influential employees, to model the behavior more frequently? If they do, you can rest assured that others will follow.

In closing, be a food safety role model and look for ways to help others do the same. Remember, role models are highly influential, whether for good or bad. If your organization does not have an ample supply of people demonstrating food safety the right way every day, the effects on non-compliance will be potent, and there may be little you can do to train or inspect your way to greater compliance.

Conclusion

My goal in this book was to provide you with a collection of some of the most interesting behavioral and social science studies I've reviewed over the past few years, which I believe have relevance to food safety.

While the 30 chapters I presented were all different, they were all similar in one respect. They were intended to provide you with new ideas and concepts that have not been thoroughly reviewed, researched, and, more importantly, applied in the field of food safety.

Remember, despite the fact that thousands of employees have been trained in food safety around the world, millions of dollars have been spent globally on food safety research, and countless inspections and tests have been performed at home and abroad, food safety remains a significant public health challenge. Why is that? I believe it's because we, as food safety professionals, need to include additional tools in our toolbox, besides the traditional tools of training, inspections, and testing.

This book was my attempt to arm you with new behavioral science tools to further improve your effectiveness at reducing food safety risks in certain parts of the food system and world, as I am convinced that we need to adopt new, out-of-the-box thinking that is more heavily focused on influencing and changing human behavior in order to accomplish this goal.

In closing, thanks for again for taking the time to read *Food Safety = Behavior* and, more importantly, for all that you are doing to advance food safety, so that people worldwide can live better.

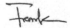

© Springer Science+Business Media New York 2015
F. Yiannas, *Food Safety = Behavior*, Food Microbiology and Food Safety,
DOI 10.1007/978-1-4939-2489-9

If you have any questions, comments, or suggestions, I would love to hear from you. You can e-mail me at foodsafetyculture@msn.com or follow me on twitter @ frankyiannas.

****

www.foodsafetyculture.com

Acknowledgment

I want to thank Nathan Jarvis for his assistance in helping me research and gather content for this book. Nathan is a bright young professional who began his career in the Hospitality industry working in restaurants, catering, and retail. After teaching food production and operations at the College of Hotel and Restaurant Management at the University of Houston, he is now pursuing a Ph.D. in food microbiology at the University of Arkansas.

Nathan spent countless hours scouring the literature and helping me find proven behavioral science studies that were relevant, interesting, and powerful. With a strong passion for all things related to food, drink, and hospitality, his help not only accelerated the completion of this book, but certainly made it a better end product.

I also need to express my gratitude to Tim Anglea for his review and edits in the book. Tim received his Master's degree in History from Clemson University in 2014. He is currently working towards his Ph.D. in History at the University of Arkansas. His research interests include Margaret Thatcher's foreign policy and Anglo-American relations. He and his wife Britney live in Rogers, Arkansas.

Thank you Nathan and Tim!

© Springer Science+Business Media New York 2015
F. Yiannas, *Food Safety = Behavior*, Food Microbiology and Food Safety,
DOI 10.1007/978-1-4939-2489-9

References

Adam H, Galinsky AD (2012) Enclothed cognition. J Exp Soc Psychol 48:918–925

Asch SE (1951) Effects of group pressure on the modification and distortion of judgments. In: Guetzkow H (ed) Groups, leadership and men. Carnegie Press, Pittsburgh, pp 177–190

Blankenship KL, Wegener D, Murray RA (2012) Circumventing resistance: using values to indirectly change attitudes. J Pers Soc Psychol 103:606–621

Brodsky W, Slor Z (2013) Background music as a risk factor for distraction among young-novice drivers. Accid Anal Prev 59:382–393

Bryan CJ, Walton GM, Rogers T, Dweck CS (2011) Motivating voter turnout by invoking the self. Proc Natl Acad Sci U S A 108(31):12653–12656

Carver CS, Scheier MF (1998) On the self-regulation of behavior. Cambridge University Press, New York

Centola D (2011) An experimental study of homophily in the adoption of health behavior. Science 334:1269–1272

Cialdini RB (1993) Influence: the psychology of persuasion. Revised edn. William Morrow and Company, Inc, New York

Chandler JJ, Pronin E (2012) Fast thought induces risk taking. Psychol Sci 23:370–374

Christakis N, Fowler J (2009) Connected, the surprising power of our social networks and how they shape our lives. Hachette Book Group, New York

Daniels AC (1999) Bringing out the best in people: how to apply the astonishing power of positive reinforcement. McGraw-Hill, New York

Degani A, Wiener E (1993) Cockpit checklists: concepts, design, and use. Hum Factors 35(2):345–359

Evans FB (1963) Selling as a dyadic relationship: a new approach. Am Behav Sci 6:76–79

Flynn FJ, Bohns V (2010) Can you do me a favor? Limitations of the commitment and consistency principle in soliciting help. Unpublished manuscript

Freedman JL, Fraser SC (1966) Compliance without pressure: the foot-in-the-door technique. J Pers Soc Psychol 4:195–202

Gasser M, Boeke J, Haffernan M, Tan R (2005) The influence of font type on information recall. N Am J Psychol 7:181–188

Gawande A (2009) The checklist manifesto: how to get things right. Metropolitan Books, Henry Holt & Company, New York

Guéguen N (2012) The sweet smell of implicit helping: effects of pleasant ambient fragrance on spontaneous help in shopping malls. J Soc Psychol 152:397–400

© Springer Science+Business Media New York 2015   113
F. Yiannas, *Food Safety = Behavior*, Food Microbiology and Food Safety,
DOI 10.1007/978-1-4939-2489-9

Janz NK, Champion VL, Strecher VJ (2002) The health belief model. In: Glanz K, Lewis FM, Rimer BK (eds) Health behavior and health education: theory, research, and practice, 3rd edn. Jossey-Bass, San Francisco, pp 45–66

Joung W, Hesketh B, Neal A (2006) "War Stories" to train for adaptive performance: is it better to learn from error or success? Appl Psychol 55(2):282–302

Keizer K, Lindenberg S, Steg L (2008) The spreading of disorder. Science 322(12):1681–1685

Langer EJ, Blank A, Chanowitz B (1978) The mindlessness of ostensibly thoughtful action: the role of "placebic" information in interpersonal interaction. J Pers Soc Psychol 36(6):635–642

Lankford MG, Zembower TR, Trick WE, Hacek DM, Noskin GA, Peterson LR (2003) Influence of role models and hospital design on hand hygiene of health care workers. Emerg Infect Dis 9(2):217–223

Lapinski MK, Maloney EK, Braz M, Shulman HC (2013) Testing the effects of social norms and behavioral privacy on hand washing: a field experiment. Hum Commun Res 39(1):21–46

Latané B, Darley J (1968) Bystander intervention in emergencies: diffusion of responsibility. J Pers Soc Psychol 8:377–383

Latané B, Darley J (1969) Bystander "Apathy". Am Sci 57:244–268

Levy M, Weitz B (1998) Retail management, 3rd edn. McGraw Hill Publishing Company, Boston

Logeswaran N, Bhattacharya J (2009) Crossmodal transfer of emotion by music. Neurosci Lett 455(2):129–133

Madesen CH, Jr. Madsen CR (1974) Teaching and discipline: behavior principles toward a positive approach. Boston: Allyn & Bacon

McGlone MS, Tofighbakhsh J (2000) Birds of a feather flock conjointly (?): rhyme as reason in aphorisms. Psychol Sci 11(5):424–428

McPherson M, Smith-Lovin L, Cook JM (2001) Birds of a feather: homophily in social networks. Ann Rev Sociol 27:415–444

Milgram S, Bickman L, Berkowitz L (1969) Note on the drawing power of crowds of different size. J Pers Soc Psychol 13(1):79–82

Murphy D (1947) How plain talk increases readership 45% to 60%. Printer's Ink 220:35–37

Naquin CE, Kurtzberg TR, Belkin LY (2010) The finer points of lying online: email versus pen and paper. J Appl Psychol 95(2):387–394

Nunes JC, Drèze X (2006) The endowed progress effect: how artificial advancement increases effort. J Consum Res 32:504–512

Olson R, Grosshuesch A, Schmidt S, Gray M, Wipfli B (2009) Observational learning and work-place safety: the effects of viewing the collective behavior of multiple social models on the use of personal protective equipment. J Safety Res 40:383–387

Ringelmann M (1913) Recherces sur les moteurs animes: Travail de l'homme (Research on animate sources of power: the work of man). Annales de l'Institut National Agronomique, 2nd series 12:1–40

Slovic P (1991) Beyond numbers: a broader perspective on the risk perception and risk communication. In: Mayo DG, Hollander RD (eds) Acceptable evidence: science and values in risk management. Oxford University Press, New York, pp 48–65

Small DA, Lowenstein G (2003) Helping a victim or helping the victim: altruism and identifiability. J Risk Uncertain 26(1):5–16

Small DA, Loewenstein G, Slovic P (2007) Sympathy and callousness: the impact of deliberative thought on donations to identifiable and statistical victims. Organ Behav Hum Decis Process 102:143–153

Song H, Schwarz N (2008) If it's hard to read, it's hard to do: processing fluency affects effort prediction and motivation. Psychol Sci 19(10):986–988

Song H, Schwarz N (2009) If it's difficult to pronounce, it must be risky: fluency, familiarity, and risk perception. Psychol Sci 20(2):135–138

The Fun Theory. The world's deepest bin. A Volkswagen initiative. http://www.youtube.com/watch?v=cbEKAwCoCKw&feature=player_embedded. Accessed 21 Sept 2001

Toma C, Hancock JT (2012) What lies beneath: the linguistic traces of deception in online dating profiles. J Commun 62:78–97

Veer R, Rank T (2012) Warning! The following packet contains graphic images: the impact of mortality salience on the effectiveness of graphic cigarette warning labels. J Consum Behav 11:225–233

Wilson J, Kelling G (1982) Broken windows. The Atlantic online. March. http://www.theatlantic.com/magazine/archive/1982/03/broken-windows/304465/

Wu D, DiGiacomo A, Kingstone A (2013) A sustainable building promotes pro-environmental behavior: an observational study on food disposal. PLoS One 8:1–4

Zhong C, Bohns VK, Gino F (2010) Good lamps are the best police: darkness increases dishonesty and self-interested behavior. Psychol Sci 21:311–314

Printed in the United States
By Bookmasters

Printed in the United States
By Bookmasters